ESSENTIALS

THE CARE PROCESS

Assessment, Planning, Implementation and Evaluation in Healthcare

MEL NEWTON, ANNE LLEWELLYN AND SALLY HAYES

Lantern

ISBN: 9781908625632

This book is an updated and revised version of *The Care Process: assessment, planning, implementation and evaluation in health and social care* by Sally Hayes and Anne Llewellyn, published in 2010 by Reflect Press Ltd (ISBN 9781906052225)

Lantern Publishing Ltd, The Old Hayloft, Vantage Business Park, Bloxham Rd, Banbury, OX16 9UX, UK
www.lanternpublishing.com

www.cla.co.uk

British Library Cataloguing in Publication Data
A catalogue record for this book is available from the British Library

The authors and publisher have made every attempt to ensure the content of this book is up to date and accurate. However, healthcare knowledge and information is changing all the time so the reader is advised to double-check any information in this text on drug usage, treatment procedures, the use of equipment, etc. to confirm that it complies with the latest safety recommendations, standards of practice and legislation, as well as local Trust policies and procedures. Students are advised to check with their tutor and/or practice supervisor before carrying out any of the procedures in this textbook.

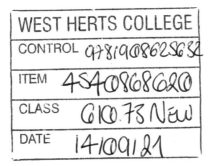
Cover design by Andrew Magee Design Ltd
Cover image reproduced under licence from stock.adobe.com

Typeset by Medlar Publishing Solutions Pvt Ltd, India
Printed in the UK

Last digit is the print number: 10 9 8 7 6 5 4 3 2

Contents

About the authors

Mel Newton is a Senior Lecturer in the School of Health and Social Care at Teesside University. She has worked for many years within the Nursing Department teaching across pre-registration and post-registration courses, but recently moved to teach leadership and human factors/patient safety. She is course Leader for MSc Human Factors and Patient Safety which is an online course.

Mel is currently undertaking a Doctorate in Professional Practice and intends to contribute to research by using ethnography to understand the healthcare culture and management of patient falls. She was awarded Senior Fellow of the HEA and enjoys student contact and learning-related activities.

Dr Anne Llewellyn is currently Deputy Director (Learning Development), Student and Library Services at Teesside University. She started working life as a Registered Nurse, and has worked in Higher Education for over 25 years, primarily in academic roles. She has been in her current post in professional services for just over one year and has responsibility for learning skills development, disability and mental health services, customer services and learning spaces.

Anne has a particular interest in enhancing the student learning experience through provision of appropriate information, support and empowerment through the use of multimedia formats that students can access at point of need. She completed her Professional Doctorate in April 2018, where she analysed the use of immersive learning spaces to enhance professional skills development, and is using this learning to inform developments to support academic and transferable skills and student digital literacy. Anne has taken on various leadership roles in higher education and was awarded Principal Fellow of the HEA in 2015 and University Teaching Fellowship in 2016.

Dr Sally Hayes is currently Director of Students at the Open University. Her academic career began at Leeds Metropolitan University where she gained experience of working with students at different academic levels within nursing and other health-related professions across pre- and post-registration education. She is particularly interested in facilitating the development of all learners, be they students of different disciplines, clinical practitioners or educationalists who base their practice on a journey of lifelong learning through critical reflection. She completed her Doctorate in 2013 which examined educational standards in nursing and is currently preparing a portfolio submission for the Principal Fellow of the Higher Education Academy.

Acknowledgements

We would firstly and most wholeheartedly like to give our thanks to the real Frank and Lizzie, who will remain anonymous but to whom we owe a debt of gratitude for the inspiration we needed to bring this book to life. Thanks also to our students, who continue to inspire us to be the best we can in supporting them to be the best they can!

Introduction

The content, coverage and approach of this book

This concise textbook is intended as an introductory text, which focuses on fundamental principles and practice of the care process for nursing students, health support workers and nursing associates. It is set out as a workbook, using case narratives to stimulate reflective learning and ground theoretical perspectives. The book can therefore be used as an independent study tool or as a core text within a particular module.

One way of conceptualising the care process is demonstrated by Sutton (2006), who uses the acronym ASPIRE to identify the different elements within the care process. Despite being published almost two decades ago, this model remains highly relevant:

- **AS**sessment
- **P**lanning
- **I**mplementation
- **R**eview and **E**valuation.

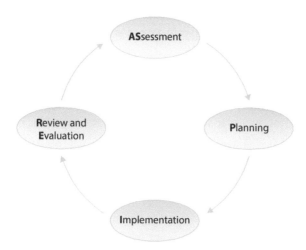

Diagrammatic representation of the cyclical process of care.

This is a cyclical and continuous process in which needs are assessed and reassessed according to ongoing evaluation. The process requires addressing a number of questions in order to undertake an assessment of need and to gather the information required to plan care and interventions. Essentially, nursing practice involves problem-solving and identifying solutions to problems, whether the individual is admitted to hospital for a short-planned operation, or receives time-limited care within the primary care sector, or they have longer-term health and/or social care needs. The care process involves a series of stages and good assessment is essential for the identification of the problem as well as setting goals and planning interventions. If we fail to assess properly, there is a risk of basing interventions on guesswork or adopting a ritualised approach to the care process.

You will be familiar with this process from other areas of our lives where we may adopt this cyclical approach to decision-making in relation to more mundane activities than providing nursing care. Imagine, for example, you are planning a visit to a friend in hospital in a distant place. You will follow a process, which includes the need to assess, plan, implement and evaluate. In the assessment, the relevant factors may be:

- Where is the hospital and how long will it take to get there and visit your friend?
- What method of transport will be the best to use and what time can you visit?
- Do you need to let her or her family know you will be visiting?
- Are there practical things you need to consider such as child care or accommodation to enable you to visit?

You will need to consider issues of finance and available resources. Planning will therefore involve matching the resources to the available options, planning the method of transport to be used and timings. All of these factors will depend on available budget and personal preferences. Implementation will focus on the visit itself and, although there may not be a formal evaluation, consideration of how it went, what worked well and what did not will influence whether you would use the same approach for a future visit.

Professional standards for nursing care and the influence of policy

The importance of this systematic and cyclical approach to care for nursing practice is demonstrated in the professional requirements for competency and proficiency.

The Nursing and Midwifery Council (NMC) governs registration for professional practice and the progression to nursing branch programmes. This body sets the standards of conduct and for the assessment and establishment of professional competency. The expected conduct of registered nurses is set out in *The Code: professional standards of practice and behaviour for nurses, midwives and nursing associates* (NMC, 2018a) and organised into four expectations:

- Prioritise people
- Practise effectively
- Preserve safety
- Promote professionalism and trust.

Throughout the book there are examples in each chapter of how your practice can be developed to meet these expectations.

Standards or proficiencies are set out and focus on the cyclical process of care delivery and, as such, require nurses to demonstrate competence in the assessment, planning and implementation of nursing care within ethical, legal and policy frameworks.

In 2017, the Nursing and Midwifery Council (NMC) consulted on and updated their Standards of Proficiency for Registered Nurses that were then introduced in January 2019. These proficiencies are required for entry to the register, enabling registrants to practise as qualified practitioners. The proficiencies are grouped under seven 'platforms' which focus on the holistic needs of service users and identify achievement of learning outcomes in relation to (NMC, 2018b):

- Being an accountable professional
- Promoting health and preventing ill health
- Assessing needs and planning care
- Providing and evaluating care
- Leading and managing nursing care and working in teams
- Improving safety and quality of care
- Coordinating care.

Running alongside the wider professional context and process of ASPIRE it is important to recognise the policy (political) context of healthcare. Policy is set by the Department of Health and essentially sets national strategy and overall direction for the NHS. Policy is important to the ASPIRE process as it influences the work of health and social care practitioners at all levels. For example, policy impacts on diverse areas of practice from the amount of resources that are available to fund (or not fund) a service, to the types of practitioners that are legally enabled or 'legitimised' to undertake certain tasks and roles.

Our approach

The book has been designed to support and extend students' learning, introducing key concepts in relation to this ASPIRE process. Each chapter has clearly defined learning outcomes and a guide to further learning. A case study of Frank and Lizzie is employed throughout the book, as this represents a complex but not atypical case that will help you to apply the theoretical aspects of the ASPIRE framework to practice. This case is based on a real case study (see below) and both Frank and Lizzie and their next of kin have given informed consent for it to be used. Some biographical details have been changed (including names) to protect anonymity, but the care elements are based on fact.

Other case studies are also used throughout the book to demonstrate the breadth of patients and service user groups that nurses encounter. These are fictional, although some elements of them may be derived from real situations to ensure authenticity. The biographical data and details of locations are all fictional and any resemblance to reality is accidental and coincidental. Throughout the book, you will also find structured activities linked to the case studies to engage the reader and help them to understand relevance to their practice.

Meet Frank and Lizzie

Frank and Lizzie are both 83 and have been happily married for 61 years. They live in a two-bedroomed bungalow on the outskirts of a small town and until recently have lived very independently.

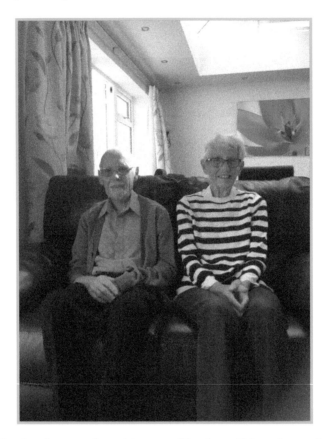

Frank left school at the age of 14 with no qualifications. Although not diagnosed at the time, he is profoundly dyslexic and still has great difficulty reading and writing. However, he has always been extremely practical, and he built their summerhouse as well as fitting the kitchen and bathroom. Throughout his life Frank has had a number of jobs, including farm worker, milkman and taxi driver. Lizzie has worked as a nurse as well as supporting Frank in their taxi business. As committed Salvationists, they ran a homeless shelter for the Salvation Army for a period of time and Frank ended his career as a prison chaplain working with young offenders. He formally retired from this role when he was 80.

Frank and Lizzie have always worked hard together to provide for their four children as well as disadvantaged people in the community. They have one son and three daughters, all of whom now have families of their own. Their son is their eldest child and lives some distance away, although he is in regular contact with them and visits them when he can. Their eldest daughter lives about 5 miles away and they see her regularly. She provides a lot of support, including helping them with their shopping and cleaning. Their middle daughter also lives fairly locally to them, but they see little of her. Their youngest child lives some distance away, but is also in regular contact and visits at least once a month.

Not long ago, Lizzie broke her ankle and shortly afterwards suffered a detached retina. This has affected her confidence and she has become increasingly dependent on Frank. She enjoyed reading and walking the dog, but since the death of their beloved Yorkshire terrier, she has become progressively less mobile and now has frequent falls. She lacks confidence socially and has always been forgetful, but over the last year her memory has dramatically deteriorated and she now has difficulty making decisions.

Frank enjoyed good health until three years ago, when he was diagnosed with Parkinson's disease and early-stage dementia. At the age of 81 he had to give up driving due to the tremors associated with his Parkinson's disease, which has impacted greatly on Frank and Lizzie's ability to be independent – they have become increasingly reliant on their eldest daughter to take them shopping and to appointments.

Last year, Frank was diagnosed with skin cancer and had a tumour removed from his face. However, the cancer spread and six months later he had to have a large tumour removed from his neck, which resulted in some nerve damage, leaving him with partial paralysis of one side of his face. This has particularly affected his mouth and his ability to eat, drink and talk. He has had courses of both radiotherapy and chemotherapy and has had further tumours removed from his scalp. Pre-operatively, he had to have a number of teeth removed and he now has dentures, which make his mouth sore. He has been deaf for some years and wears hearing aids in both ears.

Over the last year, Frank's tremors have got significantly worse and he now finds it difficult to hold anything and struggles to cut food and get it into his mouth. In addition, the paralysis of his mouth has led to problems with dribbling, which is a constant source of embarrassment for Frank. He has lost a lot of weight and looks malnourished and frail.

Lizzie worries about the future and how they will cope. Their lives have changed dramatically. They can no longer get out to the local town because Frank can't drive. Frank doesn't enjoy reading because of his dyslexia, and although Lizzie was once an avid reader, she no longer has the concentration to read a book. Frank's garden was his pride and joy, but he is no longer able to tend it due to his difficulty in holding implements and making fine motor movements. They still attend Salvation Army services when they can get someone to pick them up, but no longer feel able to play the active role that has always been a fundamental part of their lives.

In *Appendix 3* you will find a Single Assessment Process form completed for Frank as an example (see also *Chapter 4*).

Chapter outlines

Chapter 1 sets the scene by exploring definitions of health, exploring health behaviours and examining elements of the historical development of health and social care with reference to the biomedical and social models of healthcare. The chapter considers the importance of user and carer perspectives in health and social care delivery, exploring the concept of power within these relationships. This traces the origins of why the care process looks as it does by examining the role of the individuals and their specific roles as 'service user', 'carer' or 'professional practitioner'. The relationship between health and social care is also scrutinised, emphasising the importance of joint working between health and social care agencies in the provision of holistic person-centred care.

We make reference to politics and key policy drivers in health and social care, exploring the factors that influence policy and policy-making including the increasing focus on quality and the important issues about resources and finance and issues such as personalisation, risk and safeguarding. An understanding of the policy context is essential in understanding the care process, because it dictates the very manner in which ASPIRE is undertaken through funding and the establishment of national, regional and local policy targets and standards.

Communication and decision-making underpin all stages of the ASPIRE process and are discussed in *Chapters 2* and *3*, respectively. *Chapters 4* to *7* then explore the important skills used to undertake the process of care through consideration of the four-stepped process of ASPIRE – Assessment, Planning, Implementation, and Review and Evaluation. Finally, *Chapter 8* concludes the discussion by considering the future context of, and challenges for, your nursing practice.

Chapter 1
The context of nursing care

LEARNING OUTCOMES

This chapter covers the following key issues:

- Definitions of health and health behaviours

- The historical development of health (and social) care

- The importance of user and carer perspectives in care delivery

- The ways that policy affects the process of ASPIRE in health and social care.

By the end of this chapter you should be able to:

- explain what is meant by a biomedical approach to healthcare

- explain the key elements of a social model of healthcare

- engage with debates about the relationship between health and social care for personal wellbeing

- understand why policy is so important to the care process

- relate this learning to the stars of our case study – Frank and Lizzie.

While many elements of the NMC platforms that make up the standards of proficiency for registered nurses are covered, this chapter has particular reference to (NMC, 2018b):

- Platform 2: Promoting health and preventing ill health

- Platform 7: Coordinating care

For further detailed mapping please see *Appendix 1* – Detailed mapping to *Future Nurse: standards of proficiency for registered nurses*.

1.1 Introduction

Health and social care services take place within a political and ideological context that is constantly evolving. This chapter is about understanding 'needs' – how people define their own health and wellbeing needs, how 'needs' have been defined and addressed by society, and how the political context of our society therefore determines how healthcare is framed and delivered. The ASPIRE process is defined by the contemporary definition of health and social care need.

In the British political system of government, politicians (along with their advisors) set out policy proposals that are based on the political values and ideology of their political party; these are then put forward in election manifestos. These political programmes are democratically put to the electorate and the political party whose programme is supported by the majority of the population who voted forms a government. Once in power the party sets out its legislative programme and then a formal process of consultation occurs in which pressure groups can lobby for their views to be incorporated. The final detailed proposals are then set out in a 'White Paper' and there is a final parliamentary debate, following which the House of Commons votes and an Act of Parliament (legislation) is then passed.

With constantly changing policies, laws and processes in response to changing demands and ideas about how best to provide for these, health (and social) care is a dynamic area of activity. The factors influencing health (and social care) provision can be summarised using the acronym PEST (see *Figure 1.1*), which stands for **P**olitical, **E**conomic, **S**ocial and **T**echnological.

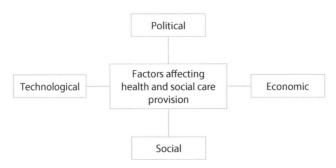

Figure 1.1 *Diagrammatic representation of the PEST acronym.*

- **Political**. This refers to the political decisions about how care should be provided. Since the early 2000s policy has emphasised a needs-led service, rather than service-led provision, with the aim of maximising independence and promoting wellbeing.
- **Economic**. This refers to the decisions about how to fund healthcare provision. Demographic changes and other factors such as globalisation and advances in pharmaceuticals mean that the cost of provision has risen, leading to the need for more efficient and cost-effective services.
- **Social**. This refers to a range of social factors that influence healthcare needs, including demographics (e.g. the age structure of the population), employment and unemployment, and lifestyle choices. In addition, the social model of healthcare has been influential in determining policy (see below).

■ **Technological**. The ever-increasing use of technology manifests itself in health and social care through the emphasis on high-tech care and intensive home care, fundamentally altering the service user journey and the role of hospital and other institutional care. In addition, developments in ICT have far-reaching implications for record-keeping (see *Chapter 6*) as well as providing greater independence for service users.

The nature of healthcare is transforming to reflect contemporary trends of population growth, demographic changes and increased public expectations about their needs and how services can be used to address these needs. When the NHS was established in 1948 to manage the illness and disease burden of society (Klein, 2005), hospital-based care was central to the organisation of healthcare services. The challenge for the NHS as a service that is expected to 'cure all ills' and meet the demand of high public expectation within finite capacity is huge, however. For example, we have many more individuals living with complex long-term conditions than we did in 1948, a challenge arising from the NHS's own success in helping to increase life expectancy.

There is tension between finite resources and seemingly ever-escalating demand (see, for example, The King's Fund 'The NHS at 70' series www.kingsfund.org.uk/publications). It could be argued, therefore, that there has been a growing mismatch between the health needs of the population and the organisation of healthcare services throughout the second half of the twentieth century.

Transformations in morbidity and mortality, public expectation and the increasing blurring of the boundaries between health and social care have led to a proposed fundamental reorganisation of services in the twenty-first century (Department of Health, 2014b). This is a complex mix of our expectations, political ideology and all the factors reflected within PEST, but also our ideas as a society and individuals about what health is and how the NHS should be prioritising its resources.

Nettleton (2013) has summarised the changing context and approach in health and social care as shown in *Table 1.1*, demonstrating questions about how we should conceptualise our focus around disease or health, be hospital or community focused and our decision to focus on cure or prevention:

Table 1.1 *Summary of changes in health and social care*

Disease	→	Health
Hospital	→	Community
Acute	→	Chronic
Cure	→	Prevention
Intervention	→	Monitoring
Treatment	→	Care
Patient	→	Person

ACTIVITY 1.1

Before reading *Section 1.2*, think about what health means to you.

What makes you decide that you feel healthy?

What makes you decide that you are unhealthy?

How might this differ if you were an elite athlete, or someone living with chronic obstructive pulmonary disease?

1.2 Defining health

Although the terms 'health' and 'healthy' are widely used in common speech and in health and social care environments, these terms are rather complex and difficult to define. In 1990 the Health and Lifestyles survey was carried out by a multidisciplinary group of researchers to explore lay people's perceptions and views about health (Blaxter, 2010). They identified a number of different subjective definitions of health, which incorporated medical, social and holistic elements (*Table 1.2*).

Table 1.2 *Lay definitions of health (source: Blaxter (1990) Health and Lifestyles, Chapter 2)*

Definition of health	Sample response
As not ill	Someone I know who is very healthy is me, because I haven't been to a doctor yet
Despite disease	I am very healthy despite this arthritis
As a reserve	Both parents are still alive at 90 so he belongs to healthy stock
As 'the healthy life'	I call her healthy because she goes jogging and doesn't eat fried food
As physical fitness	There's tone to my body, I feel fit
As energy or vitality	Health is when I feel I can do anything
As social relationships	You feel as though everyone is your friend, I enjoy life more, and can work, and help other people
As function	She's 81 and she gets her work done quicker than me, and she does the garden
As psychosocial wellbeing	Well I think health is when you feel happy

Health is thus defined in many different ways. To explore these definitions of health and their theoretical bases, we can broadly divide the definitions of health into three sub-categories:

1. The biomedical definition (the absence of disease model of health).
2. Social models of health, which see health as a social phenomenon.

3. Holistic models, which view health as determined by psychosocial, biological, environmental and spiritual factors (considered in more detail at the end of this chapter).

1.2.1 The biomedical approach to health and illness

The absence of disease model of health and illness is based on the medical model of healthcare, which has dominated formal healthcare delivery in the Western world since the eighteenth century. This model developed as part of a wider social process of scientific development. It replaced previous unscientific explanations of health and illness, which viewed ill health either as an imbalance with the natural world, a punishment from an external force or being (such as a supernatural being), or based on the miasmic theory, where illness was viewed as the result of bad smells (Hayes and Llewellyn, 2008). The biomedical model of illness is based on five assumptions:

1. **The mechanical metaphor of the body** – the body can be broken down into component parts, and these component parts can be isolated and the dysfunctions treated, similar to the analogy of car maintenance and repair.
2. **Mind–body dualism** – the mind and body are seen as separate from one another, and therefore do not have any influence on each other.
3. **The doctrine of specific aetiology** – or cause and symptoms. Specific causes can be identified and treated for each disease.
4. **The technological imperative** – the merits and benefits of technological interventions (either through surgical and other invasive procedures or through pharmacological prescriptions) are valued.
5. **Reductionism** – the model reduces individuals to a set of anatomical and physiological processes, with lesser emphasis on psychosocial and environmental processes.

Within this model then, health is equated with absence of disease and needs are assessed in terms of those factors that need to be addressed to rid the individual of disease or illness. For example, an individual who has hypothermia needs to have their core body temperature increased slowly until it returns to normal parameters.

FRANK AND LIZZIE

If we apply this to the case study of Frank and Lizzie, we can see that Frank has specific diagnoses of Parkinson's disease, malignant tumours and early-stage dementia (specific aetiology). He takes a range of medications and has had surgery to remove malignant tumours (technological imperative). Frank sees a number of doctors for his different diagnoses, which reflects the mechanical metaphor and reductionist nature of his treatments, with a focus on managing the physical symptoms of his memory loss, tremors and mobility problems (mind–body dualism).

1.2.2 Social models of health

In the 1960s, the discipline of medical sociology developed as a sub-discipline of sociology. Medical sociologists not only questioned the validity and objectivity of the medical model of healthcare (Illich, 1976), but also proposed a social model to explain health and illness. Social models generally have three characteristics:

1. Health and illness are produced within a social context, influencing how people interpret and experience health and illness.
2. Social variables are important determinants of health and illness. While the biomedical model sees health and illness as a natural process, the social model acknowledges that social factors influence the biological processes. Thus, social variables such as class, gender, ethnicity and geographical location all impact on both disease and illness causation. Using the example of hypothermia above, the individual would not only need to have their core body temperature increased, but there would also be a need to assess the social factors that may have contributed to hypothermia – for example, whether their house is adequately heated, whether they have sufficient income to use heating, whether they have sufficient warm clothing.
3. Healthcare is not objective, but decisions are made based on people's personal characteristics. For example, there are differences in the way that men and women are diagnosed and treated based on gender stereotypes.

Understanding the subjective interpretation of health and illness is important when assessing and planning care, as it may impact on issues such as assessment of the need for professional involvement, compliance with planned interventions (for example, drug regimens) and self-assessment of needs. These issues will be discussed in more detail later in this chapter.

ACTIVITY 1.2

Have a look at the following website created by The Health Foundation, and identify the social variables that impact on health and illness: www.health.org.uk/blog/infographic-what-makes-us-healthy

---

The social model of health and social care has also been increasingly influential in determining policy. This emerged through the disability rights movement, arguing for increased control over services and the determination of need, and has subsequently spread to other service user groups. This has led to a much greater emphasis on empowerment and user-led services and will be drawn out further in our discussions related to the concept of 'wellbeing'.

1.2.3 The functionalist approach to health

The work of Talcott Parsons (1951) has been particularly influential in identifying the social as well as biological basis of illness (Hayes and Llewellyn, 2008) (*Table 1.3*). Parsons was a functionalist sociologist, believing that society is made up not just of individuals and their actions, but also of a series of interdependent systems and structures. The smooth running of society is dependent on individuals and these systems operating in harmony to maintain the status quo. Thus functionalists are interested in the roles that people have and how these roles and responsibilities are managed for the collective good.

Table 1.3 *Summary of the differences between the medical model and the social model of healthcare (Moon and Gillespie, 1995)*

Medical model	Social model
A state of health is a biological fact: it is immutable, real, independent.	A state of health is socially constructed: it is varied, uncertain, diverse.
Ill health is caused by biological calamities: • 'entrants' to the body (e.g. viruses, germs) • 'internal faults' (e.g. genes) • trauma	Ill health is caused by social factors: • behind the biology lies society • root causes are social causes
Causes are identified by: • signs and symptoms • the process of 'diagnosis' • from medically established 'normality'	Causes are identified through: • beliefs, which are varying, subjective, society- and community-based • interpretation, built up through custom and social constraint
Medical knowledge is exclusionary: • it is the job of the expert or specialist • facts are accumulated and built upon • alternative perspectives are invalid and inferior	Knowledge is not exclusionary: • it has a historical, cultural and social context • it is shaped by involved people
Biomedicine is reductionist and disease-oriented, concerned with pathology.	The social model is holistic and concerned with context.

For functionalists, the inability to maintain roles and responsibilities is seen as deviant, in that it disrupts the equilibrium and smooth running of society. To address this, Parsons developed the sick role concept, arguing that if people were unable to fulfil roles and responsibilities, then they should be assigned a new role, the sick role, which would exempt them from their obligations. However, these exemptions were based on obligations on the part of the sick person to get better. The sick role is based on the following exemptions and obligations:

1. Exemption from normal social responsibilities (for example, work and family roles).
2. Exemption from responsibility for own illness (i.e. the sick person cannot be expected to get better through their own free will).
3. The obligation to be motivated to get better.
4. The obligation to seek technically competent help.

Parsons sees the medical profession as the objective providers of technically competent help. Although he sees illness as a social phenomenon as well as a biological malfunction, he concurs with the dominance of the biomedical model within the formal system of healthcare, and assumes that there is a one-way relationship between patient and doctor, with the doctor holding power in terms of diagnosis, treatment and referral. This notion of personal roles and responsibilities fits with Blaxter's (2010) definition of health as function, in that health is seen as the ability to perform daily activities of living.

FRANK AND LIZZIE

If we relate this to Frank and Lizzie, we can see that Frank has increasing difficulty in carrying out functions such as eating and drinking, communicating and mobilising, whilst Lizzie also has difficulties with the functions of mobility and cognitive processing and decision-making.

Many professional models of care have focused on helping people to manage their daily activities of living, either through adaptation or rehabilitation, and have used these functions as the basis for their model of assessment. Roper, Logan and Tierney (2000) developed a model for nursing practice in 1980, which remains relevant today. This is based on 12 activities of living, which should be viewed on the independence–dependence continuum. These activities of living are:

- maintaining a safe environment
- communication
- breathing
- eating and drinking
- elimination
- washing and dressing
- controlling temperature
- mobilisation
- working and playing
- expressing sexuality
- sleeping
- death and dying.

Within this model of care, nurses are guided to assess the patient's ability to perform functions and to plan and implement a package of care to address any deficits (these issues will be developed further in *Chapters 4* to *7*). Similarly, occupational therapists use a model of activities of daily living when working to optimise individual independence (Forster *et al.*, 2009) and social workers use a systems approach when working with individuals and families (Thompson and Thompson, 2008).

1.2.4 Lay perspectives of health

Theories of health are therefore important in informing professional models of working with service users. However, lay perspectives on health are also important, as they locate health and health and illness behaviours within the context of people's individual lives and help us to understand the subjective experience of health and illness. This is increasingly important as the ASPIRE process is concerned with needs as identified by the care recipient themselves, and as self-assessment of needs becomes more central to the process of care delivery (see *Chapter 4*).

Social roles in lay definitions of health

As identified by Blaxter (1990 and 2010), social roles are important in lay definitions of health. The notions of wellbeing and social relationships are important within lay conceptualisations of health and illness, and these social concepts form an important aspect of human existence and social involvement.

Think of the different roles that you have within your family or social network. What responsibilities to other people do you have in these roles?

The impact of health and illness on social relationships and roles is based on subjective assessment, as individuals locate health and illness within the context of their own lives and belief and value systems. This personal assessment of health is known as a lay health belief, based on social factors as opposed to the medical model of health, which is seen as a professional model of health belief, based on objective and measurable criteria. Lay health beliefs are determined by a complex set of social factors, and are individual and unique, as opposed to the universal assumptions about health within the medical model.

Lay definitions of health are therefore:
- located within social environments and contexts
- influenced by social factors such as
    - class
    - gender
    - ethnicity
    - location in social structures
    - personal experiences
    - peers
    - education system
    - mass media
    - health professionals.

Family also plays a significant role in shaping early perceptions and beliefs about health and illness. Sociologists see the family as an important unit of primary socialisation, where behaviours and beliefs are shaped (see, for example, Llewellyn *et al.*, 2015).

Think about your own definition of health. How has this been influenced by behaviours learned within your family?

1.3 **Social needs**

Social needs are much more difficult to define than health needs and it is difficult to separate health needs from social needs. There is a subjective element to the identification of needs, and there may be little agreement between individuals as to what constitutes a need.

Make a list of ten needs.
- Is there a pattern of logic in the list of needs you have drawn up?
- Do some needs come before others?
- Are some needs more basic or fundamental?
- Is your list culture-free?
- Which of these needs would you define as health needs?
- Which of these needs would you define as social needs?

Social needs can be defined in a number of ways:
- **Felt needs** – individuals are conscious of their needs (Bradshaw, 1972), which incorporates a subjective element of interpretation. For example, an individual may feel that they need to be referred for physiotherapy to start to walk and exercise safely again.
- **Expressed needs** – these are needs that are publicised and as these needs are known about, they can become demands. For example, media stories identifying the availability (often referred to as 'rationing') of medicines, including new and often very costly anticancer drugs and treatments for fertility (such as IVF), give rise to an expectation that, as drugs become available, they should be accessible to all who might benefit from them. This can be amplified when such treatments are available overseas.

Find a case in the media where an expressed need has become an expectation or a demand, such as the 2015 case of Ashya King (see www.bbc.co.uk/news/uk-england-32013634).

- **Normative needs** – these are needs that are defined according to professional norms or standards, which involves the input of outside observers or experts. This model of addressing need has been historically employed within the personal social services, as welfare professionals have had responsibility for assessing needs and planning interventions.
- **Comparative needs** – these incorporate the concept of relative judgement, and can be seen in the context of eligibility criteria and the duty introduced in the Health and Social Care Act (Department of Health, 2012a) on the Secretary of State, NHS England and clinical commissioning groups to 'have regard to the need to reduce inequalities' in access to care and outcomes of care (see *Chapter 3*).

Return to the case study in the Introduction about Frank and Lizzie. Make a list of about ten of Frank and Lizzie's health and social care needs. Try to identify which of their needs are health needs and which are social needs.

This case study demonstrates the complexity of the concept of need and the overlap between health needs and social care needs. Parry-Jones and Soulsby (2001) discuss the problems of assessing need and conclude that it is essential to clarify when something is a health need or social need if health and social care agencies are to carry out their functions effectively and work collaboratively to address the service user's needs. We will return to the case study about Frank and Lizzie at points throughout the book to demonstrate the ASPIRE process in practice.

1.4 Holistic care

The World Health Organization (WHO) acknowledged the complexity of health and the interrelationship of the different elements in its 1948 definition of health:

> *The extent to which an individual or group is able, on the one hand, to realize aspirations and satisfy needs and on the other hand, to change or cope with the environment. Health is therefore seen as a resource for everyday life, not the objective of living: it is a positive concept emphasizing social and personal resources as well as physical capabilities.* (World Health Organization, 1948)

The ability to function both physically and socially is an important determinant of health. Ill health has biological and psychosocial consequences for the individual, and therefore needs to be seen within a social as well as a medical context. In addition, the social context is important in terms of illness behaviour.

It is increasingly recognised that a holistic concept, amalgamating elements of the two models, provides the most comprehensive approach to both understanding and delivering health and social care (see *Figure 1.2*). Holistic care is defined as the interrelationship between biological, psychological and social factors (Hockley and Clark, 2002); while for Patterson (1998), holistic care encompasses elements of mind, body and spirit.

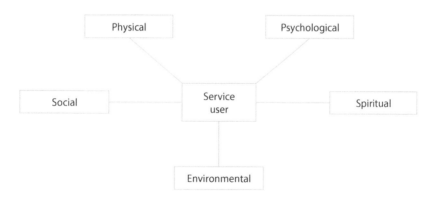

Figure 1.2 *A diagrammatic representation of holistic care.*

Health and social care are complex and multidimensional concepts and there is a need for a holistic approach to care that addresses both health and social needs, with agencies working in partnership to provide packages of care that address individual need. Services have historically developed according to a welfarist model, where welfare professionals have identified needs and then provided services to address these needs (see the discussion above about normative need). The increase in consumerism has led to greater emphasis on user and carer involvement in care and individual assessment of need and care packages tailored to meet those needs. A consumerist approach to health and illness sees care as a commodity, which can be bought and sold, leading to greater control and choice for care recipients (Glasby, 2017). There is a shift from service-led provision to needs-led care, with the care recipient at the centre of the decision-making process.

There is a much greater emphasis on 'self-help' or 'self-health', based on the ways in which people take responsibility for their own health and motivate themselves to avoid or manage illness. This can include lifestyle choices such as diet, exercise and relaxation, or healthcare choices such as complementary and alternative therapies. This reflects the greater emphasis on individual resources and how these can be used to promote wellbeing.

One example of this is the work of the government-commissioned 'What Works Centre for Wellbeing', the aim of which is to "improve, and save, lives through better policy and practice for wellbeing" (see www.whatworkswellbeing.org). Wellbeing is a complex concept but has been defined by the 'What Works Centre for Wellbeing' network as providing "a way to understand what's needed and how best we can all work together to improve our lives in a complex world. It brings together economic, social, environmental, democratic and personal outcomes and avoids focusing on specific areas at the expense of others. We can be better at measuring what matters and using what we know to create a better society. It is about engaging citizens in meaningful deliberation about what better society could look like".

This shift in ideology and balance of provision of services has led to a need for more collaborative and partnership working between the different professional groups involved in the delivery of health and social care and with service users and carers (see *Chapter 5*).

ACTIVITY 1.8

In 2007 the UK government introduced a ban on smoking in public places. This has meant that smoking is not permitted in any publicly-owned buildings or in workplaces such as pubs or residential homes.
1. Think about how the policy on smoking has impacted on the following individuals.
2. Identify the ways in which their health and social care needs are met.

Case study 1

Lizzie's older sister Ivy is 86 and has smoked for 73 years. She lives in a local authority care home and is unable to get outside independently.

Case study 2

Frank and Lizzie's neighbour Greta has brittle asthma. Before the smoking ban was introduced, she was actually frightened to go into a pub with her friends, as when she was 18 she went to the pub to celebrate and had to leave as she was having difficulty with her chest feeling tight and experiencing shortness of breath.

Case study 3

Jane is a Practice Nurse. She is an ex-smoker and since 2007 has managed a 'quit smoking' clinic that her practice established as part of the response to changes in legislation and – importantly – an increase in funding for the provision of services for individuals wanting to quit.

These very brief case studies illustrate the impact of health policy at both service and individual level. Ivy's case raises questions about how the home will address her desire to carry on smoking and ensure that they are able to meet Ivy's assessed needs in a planned way. Perhaps they may assess her and decide the best option is for Ivy to quit smoking, or the assessment of her need may be that it would be too difficult for her to quit. Could they therefore plan to provide a smoking area outside the property or would the law allow smoking inside the resident's bedroom as she lives in a residential home? There are implications of implementing either of these plans, in terms of Ivy's freedom of choice or her socialising within the day areas or the dangers of smoking in a bedroom, isolated from staff and other residents.

The case for Greta is far less contentious. Since the ban has been in place she has been able to go to her local pub in the knowledge that she will not be exposed to tobacco smoke and so getting out with her friends who like to go to the pub to socialise is now possible for her.

In terms of service provision the policy of reducing smoking in the population as a whole is a great relief to Jane. She had tried unsuccessfully through the 1990s to set up a 'quit smoking' clinic but now, due to increased funding for smoking cessation services, she can access funding to run a local clinic. She also has a number of services that she can refer smokers to if they prefer not to attend the GP surgery for their 'quit smoking' advice. This includes stop smoking clinics, brief intervention services, access to medication to help the addiction (patches and tablets) and there is even a 'smoke-free houses' service that will visit families to advise on keeping homes free of smoke.

These case studies demonstrate how policies affect individuals and societies and how they influence decisions about assessment, planning and implementation of care. But what is policy and who decides on which policies are introduced?

1.5 What are the driving forces behind policy direction?

There are a number of factors that drive policy direction, which demonstrate the complexity of the context of policy decisions. Examples of influencing factors include:

1.5.1 Demographics – the ageing population

Demographic changes have led to changing patterns of health and illness. Across Western societies, there is an ageing population, and although old age and ill health are not inextricably linked, there is a higher incidence of ill health and in particular, chronic and complex ill health amongst the older population. NHS spending on the 65+ age group is almost double that for the under 65s (Llewellyn *et al.*, 2015).

Significantly, although life expectancy has increased, healthy life expectancy has not risen as fast, creating greater demands on health and social care services. New factors associated with ageing that may be detrimental to health have emerged as a result of this. For example, loss and grief are significant risk factors, which disproportionately affect older people.

FRANK AND LIZZIE

If we return to the case study of Frank and Lizzie, we can see a number of loss factors that are affecting their lives. Frank has lost functional activities, related to his difficulty in making fine motor movements, reductions in his mobility and his inability to drive. Lizzie has lost some capacity to make decisions and they both have lost fundamental social relations and meaningful occupation, such as gardening and reading.

The impact of this on individuals and society is reflected in growing numbers of older people suffering from depression and taking their own lives. It is estimated that 20% of older people in the community suffer from depression and this rises to 40% of those living in care homes (Public Health England, 2017a).

In addition, while life expectancy has risen significantly in the last 50 years, the birth rate has fallen. This has significant implications for state-funded health and social care services as the current working population pays taxes to support those who have retired. There will therefore be a crisis of funding that will have huge implications for health and social care services, and policy changes regarding later retirement ages and the funding of residential and nursing care homes are currently hotly debated political issues.

ACTIVITY 1.9

1. What will be the impact of an increasing older population on the provision of health and social care services?
2. What policy decisions may the government need to make in order to ensure that health and social care services reach those who need them?

1.5.2 Social determinants of health

There is an emerging body of research exploring social determinants of health (SDH) and the implications for healthcare policy and practice. These social determinants of health include:

- poverty
- homelessness
- alcohol and drug addiction
- malnutrition (including obesity)
- environment
- lifestyle practices such as gambling, gaming and smoking
- idealised body image.

It is beyond the scope of this book to explore all of these factors in depth (see Llewellyn *et al.*, 2015, for a more detailed discussion of the social context of disadvantage across a range of service user groups), but the concept of SDH has implications for nursing care and the ASPIRE process. With the focus on holistic care, as discussed throughout this book, nursing is well placed to improve patient health through linking social factors to health outcomes in their assessments of care (Olshansky, 2017). This requires a broad understanding of the social context of health, so that nurses can ask appropriate questions about the individual's circumstances and explore whether health or community resources can be used to assist their patients. This is a fundamental aspect of contemporary healthcare and requires skills for assessing a person's social context and influences and developing planned interventions to promote good health and wellbeing.

1.5.3 Technological and pharmaceutical advances

In addition to the demographic shift that has led to older people constituting a greater proportion of the population, one of the major policy pressures is the expenditure push associated with innovations in medical technology. The key element of this is the cost of pharmaceuticals (Crinson, 2008) and as we make increasing use of novel medical technological improvements, costs will rise.

1.5.4 The rise in the incidence of long-term conditions

Such demographic changes and medical and technological advances have led to a rise in the incidence of long-term conditions (LTCs). This refers to the number of individuals living with chronic illnesses such as diabetes, heart disease and chronic obstructive pulmonary disease, which can limit lifestyle. Patients with multiple LTCs are becoming the norm rather than the exception and the number of people with comorbidities was set to increase in England from 1.9 million in 2008 to 2.9 million by 2018 (Department of Health, 2014b). This demonstrates how – although the UK population is living longer – the extra years are not necessarily spent in good health or free from illness or disability.

The difference between life expectancy and health expectancy can be regarded as an estimate of the number of years a person can expect to live in poor health or with a limiting illness or disability. In 1981 the expected time men lived in poor health was 6.5 years. By 2004 this had risen to 8.6 years. Women can expect to live longer in poor health than men. In 1981 the expected time women lived in poor health was 10.1 years, rising to 19.1 years in 2016. The time men can expect to live with a limiting illness or disability has also increased between 1981 and 2016: 12.8 years in 1981 rising to 16.1 years in 2016 (Public Health England, 2017b).

> ### ACTIVITY 1.10
>
> 1. How might the increasing complexity of needs among the ageing population impact on the assessment and planning process?
> 2. Who needs to be involved?

ACTIVITY 1.11 – THE IMPACT OF POLICY ON THE CARE OF FRANK

Refer back to the case study about Frank and Lizzie.

Reflecting on this chapter, list policies and guidance that would have impacted on the way in which the care that Frank and Lizzie needed was delivered through the ASPIRE process.

Many policies will have impacted on the care that both Lizzie and Frank received. The following are examples, although this is not an exhaustive list:

- Frank had skin cancer – National Cancer Programme (see www.gov.uk/government/publications/national-cancer-programme-bulletin-issue-21-september-2011).
- Frank is showing early signs of dementia – 'After a diagnosis of dementia: what to expect from health and care services' (see www.gov.uk/government/publications/after-a-diagnosis-of-dementia-what-to-expect-from-health-and-care-services).
- Frank has Parkinson's disease and wants to stay at home – NICE guidance for treatment and 'Comorbidities: a framework of principles for system-wide action' (see www.gov.uk/government/publications/better-care-for-people-with-2-or-more-long-term-conditions).

You may wish to visit the Department of Health and Social Care website (www.gov.uk/government/organisations/department-of-health-and-social-care) and examine more closely how it relates to the ASPIRE process.

CHAPTER SUMMARY

This chapter has explored what is meant by a biomedical approach to health and examined the key elements of a social model of healthcare. It has examined the nature of policy and its importance to the care process, drawing on the experiences of Frank and Lizzie to illustrate impact.

Reflection

Identify at least three things that you have learned from this chapter.	
	1. ....
	....
	2. ....
	....
	3. ....
	....

How do you plan to use this knowledge within clinical practice?

1. ....
....
2. ....
....
3. ....
....

How will you evaluate the effectiveness of your plan?

1. ....
....
2. ....
....
3. ....
....

What further knowledge and evidence do you need?

1. ....
....
2. ....
....
3. ....
....

Further Reading

Glasby, J. (2017) *Understanding Health and Social Care*, 3rd edition. Bristol: Policy Press.

This is a very accessible book that explores a number of the key issues that have been discussed in this chapter. There are chapters on partnership working in health and social care, independent living and the social model of disability and user involvement in health and social care. Concepts are illustrated through clear explanations supported by tables and diagrams to highlight key points, and at the end of each chapter there are some suggestions for further reading to develop understanding of the different concepts.

Nettleton, S. (2013) *The Sociology of Health and Illness*. Cambridge: Polity.

This is a well-written, engaging and theoretically-informed discussion of health sociology in modern Britain. It blends relevant classical and contemporary theories into an explanation of key concepts and issues and provides a lively, balanced, up-to-date introduction to medical sociology. It also discusses issues of interest to health economists, health services researchers and healthcare policy-makers.

The Social Care Institute for Excellence provides clear guidance on the process of personalisation in health and social care: www.scie.org.uk/personalisation/practice/nhs-staff

Crinson, I. (2008) *Health Policy: a critical perspective*. London: Sage.

This book examines developments in health and healthcare policy in the UK, covering issues such as the policy-making process, the development of the NHS, healthcare governance, health promotion, and the comparative analysis of healthcare systems within the European Union (EU) and the USA. Social and political themes are considered to draw together theory, historical detail and an interesting wider social commentary with case studies illustrating how policy has evolved and developed in recent years, and the implications these changes have for practice.

Chapter 2
Communication

LEARNING OUTCOMES

This chapter will consider communication within the assessment, planning, intervention and evaluation phases of the care process and will cover the following issues:

- The importance of communication within the ASPIRE process
- Models for communicating with service users
- Tools to aid the communication process.

By the end of this chapter, you should be able to:

- understand the importance of communication skills within ASPIRE
- identify a range of tools that can be used to aid communication with a range of service users
- develop your own communication skills and use them effectively in your care practice.

This chapter has relevance to all the proficiencies (NMC, 2018b) and is specifically relevant to Annexe A: Communication and relationship management skills:

1 Underpinning communication skills for assessing, planning, providing and managing best practice, evidence-based nursing care

2 Evidence-based, best practice approaches to communication for supporting people of all ages, their families and carers in preventing ill health and in managing their care.

2.1 Introduction

Effective communication is a fundamental part of caring practice and contributes to high-quality care as evaluated by care recipients (see *Chapter 7*). Communication is essential to all the steps of the ASPIRE process. For example, active listening is a vital part of assessment in order to fully understand the individual's needs and concerns. Planning and implementation require clear communication within the multidisciplinary team and sensitive explanation and discussion with the patient.

Interpersonal communication is used in any care situation as a planned activity to help individuals and families prevent or cope with illness or difficult experience (Hayes and Llewellyn, 2008). Purposeful communication, as used by professional carers, demonstrates planning and intention in the development of the interpersonal relationship. It involves the following steps:

- Guiding
- Planning
- Purposefully directing the interaction in order to enable individuals and in some cases empower them to find their own solutions.

Shannon and Weaver (1949) proposed a model of communication that has been used to guide professionals. This involves a process where a message is sent via a signal from a source and is received at a destination (*Figure 2.1*).

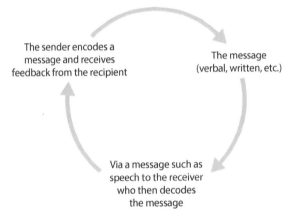

The sender encodes a message and receives feedback from the recipient

The message (verbal, written, etc.)

Via a message such as speech to the receiver who then decodes the message

Figure 2.1 *The communication loop (adapted from Glasper and Quiddington, 2009).*

ACTIVITY 2.1

Think of a very normal daily activity, such as greeting your partner or child after a day at work: "Hi, how was your day?"

Unpick the nuance of the message – 'decode' it!

How would the receiver know you are genuinely interested in their day or otherwise?

How would you know if your loved one had not had a good day, even though their words might be "Great, thank you!"?

Communication within a care encounter is a two-way process. A caring professional will not only transmit a message but will also assess the impact of that message on the receiver, who will give messages back to the sender. Healthcare practitioners are both senders and receivers of messages, using more than one strategy and signal to transmit a message, and communication is not simply about words, but includes a whole range of gestures, different sounds, facial expressions and body language.

Key principles to consider when communicating with care recipients can be explored by asking specific questions.

Think about Frank and Lizzie. You are trying to ask Lizzie about her pain levels following her fracture, or want to understand her concerns about coping with Frank's increasing frailty. These are questions you may need to consider:

- Can she hear me? Does she have a hearing aid that is working?
- Will she listen to me? Does she wear spectacles and are they clean?
- What is my non-verbal communication? Am I giving 'positive' non-verbal signals?
- Am I allowing enough time?
- Am I actively listening to Lizzie?
- What is Lizzie's story?
- Am I using open or closed questions appropriately?

2.1.1 Can they hear me?

Always ask yourself whether the recipient can 'hear' the message. This can relate to physical aspects of hearing – are they hearing-impaired, is there too much background noise, can they understand your spoken language? – or they might be so distracted (through anxiety, pain or grief, for example) that they simply cannot listen.

FRANK AND LIZZIE

In relation to Frank and Lizzie, Frank is very hard of hearing. He was fitted with new hearing aids by the audiologist at the local hospital. However, although they were made using the latest technology, the hearing aids were too small for Frank to be able to manipulate them and fit them into his ears due to his difficulties with fine motor movements. He has since had different hearing aids made that he can manipulate more easily, which has significantly improved his hearing. This demonstrates the importance of not only providing people with appropriate aids and adaptations, but also ensuring good fit and ability of usage.

In addition to ensuring that the person can hear you, using appropriate language is also very important. People may not understand what you are saying when you use medical or professional language that they do not recognise. It is important therefore to focus on the person and talk 'with' them rather than 'at' them, adopting a person-centred style (Glasper & Quiddington, 2009).

hello my name is…

The 'Hello my name is…' campaign was started by the late Dr Kate Grainger. Kate was a doctor who had cancer and needed hospital treatment, and was concerned that staff did not introduce themselves to her. This is a useful way to introduce yourself to a patient and will let you assess their communication response. By introducing yourself, you are asking to engage with the patient and the verbal and non-verbal response from the patient can be very informative. For example, looking away from you could suggest that they don't want to talk to you.

2.1.2 Will they listen to me?

Is there a reason why the care recipient may disengage? This depends on building rapport and establishing a relationship of trust that enables you to know whether the individual has understood the messages you are trying to convey and is working with you to establish a plan of action as necessary.

FRANK AND LIZZIE

In Frank and Lizzie's case there may be a number of reasons they may ignore a healthcare professional. For example:
- Lizzie: "My ankle really hurts, I wish this nurse would just stop talking and let me close my eyes for a moment."
- Frank: "What does that young thing think they are doing, asking me if I have been to the toilet today?"
- Frank: "Who are you? Why do these strangers keep coming into my house and demanding things?"

Think also about Frank's early-onset dementia. How might dementia affect his ability to concentrate, remember things or trust someone he has never met before?

There is clear guidance from the NMC Code (NMC, 2018a) concerning how we promote professionalism and trust. The code requires that nurses model integrity and leadership to ensure trust and confidence in the profession from patients, people receiving care, other healthcare professionals and the public. The code includes (among others) the following standards:
- act with honesty and integrity at all times, treating people fairly and without discrimination, bullying or harassment
- be aware at all times of how your behaviour can affect and influence the behaviour of other people
- treat people in a way that does not take advantage of their vulnerability or cause them upset or distress
- make sure you do not express your personal beliefs (including political, religious or moral beliefs) to people in an inappropriate way
- use all forms of spoken, written and digital communication (including social media and networking sites) responsibly, respecting the right to privacy of others at all times.

Appearance is also important in establishing trust and confidence. Dressing professionally and having good personal hygiene may aid the communication process. A scruffy or dirty appearance may detract from the communication process.

To determine whether a message has been understood, it is useful to ask the patient to explain back to you what has been discussed. It can be enlightening to hear what the patient has understood from your discussion. Be wary about a patient who nods to say that they have understood you. They might just want you to leave them alone or may feel embarrassed that they don't understand (see also the discussion on outpacing in *Section 2.1.4 (Table 2.1)*.

2.1.3 Am I giving the 'right' non-verbal signals?

Studies have shown that non-verbal behaviours including smiling, service user-directed eye gazing, positive head nodding, leaning forward when talking, and touch are essential (Caris-Verhallen *et al.*, 1999).

2.1.4 Am I allowing enough time?

If the individual feels rushed, they may feel undervalued and not share important information, so it is useful to communicate to the person that you have enough time or, if you do not, arrange to see the client when you do have time.

2.1.5 Am I listening to the person?

Active listening (Quilter *et al.*, 1993) is an important skill based on being sincerely attentive. It enables the listener to decode the messages they are receiving, demonstrates back to the client that you have understood them and thus establishes effective communication, which enables productive dialogue. This can be achieved through reflecting, paraphrasing and summarising, reflecting non-verbal signals and using praise.

Language is important here as well – consider an older adult asking to 'spend a penny', meaning that they want to use the toilet. If the carer is from a different cultural background or has never heard that expression before, the message may not be understood, causing distress to a person who needs to use the toilet.

2.1.6 What is the person's story?

Communication is not only about the carer's skills of communicating with the care recipients but, importantly, it is also about how the carer enables the individual to communicate their narrative. There is empirical evidence of the benefits of allowing people to talk, which contextualises their suffering within the context of their lives. This helps the carer to understand the situation from the care recipient's perspective as well as identifying resources that they may have to address the problems. Therefore, rather than being an unstructured activity, storytelling is a purposeful and planned process, based on sound empirical evidence (Fredriksson and Lindström, 2002).

2.1.7 Do I need to use open or closed questions?

Closed questions enable a simple 'yes' or 'no' answer, whereas open questions require more explanation. Sometimes it is most appropriate to limit the amount of information you need to ask for. For example, think about patients who are breathless – a question that requires a yes or no response might be most appropriate. Consider the effort needed to respond to 'Do you need to use the toilet?' as opposed to 'How can I help you?' Alternatively, closed questions can sometimes enable a person to avoid 'bothering' or worrying you.

FRANK AND LIZZIE

Think for example about Lizzie, who by nature does not want to cause a fuss. Following her fractured ankle she is likely to try to hide pain by, for example, answering a simple 'yes' to a question such as "Are you managing to control your pain?" By opening the question and saying, "I know ankles can be very painful when they are healing, what time of the day is it worst?" you may be able to find out more information from Lizzie.

2.2 Models for communicating effectively

There are various models that can help you to think about how to communicate effectively with patients. All of these models have the common goal of ensuring that the communication is as effective as possible and provide different ways of looking at how the nurse can engage with patients in order to develop the good interpersonal relationships that are essential to the ASPIRE process. In general, nurses should ensure that they are connecting with people and are using language that they understand:

- Use basic language – avoid being patronising, but think about the words that you are using. In particular, avoid using jargon, especially in terms of complex medical terminology.
- Speak at a measured pace. You need to give patients time to process what you are saying. If you speak too quickly, patients and carers may not understand what you are saying or may feel inhibited about asking questions.
- Ask the patient (and carers if relevant) questions. Teach-back is a simple process for checking understanding. To determine whether a message has been understood, it could be useful to ask the patient to explain back to you what has been discussed. It can be enlightening to hear what the patient has understood from your discussion.
- Take the time to ask the patient whether they have any questions rather than waiting for them to take the initiative. This can give the person 'permission' to ask and is an important message in validating their experiences and hearing any concerns that they may have (see discussion of invalidation in *Section 2.4 (Table 2.1)*).

Rapport is an important part of the interpersonal relationship. There are a number of models that help you to think about how you might initially approach a communication encounter with a patient.

Stickley (2011) proposes the SURETY model as an approach to a conversation. This involves the following steps:

- **S**it at an angle: this can be less threatening than sitting facing someone, which may seem like an interrogation. Sitting at an angle can help you to make eye contact, without the person feeling as though you are staring at them.
- **U**ncross legs and arms; non-verbal body language is as important as verbal messages. Crossed arms and legs can be interpreted as closed body language, making you seem less approachable.
- **R**elax: if you are relaxed, the person that you are communicating with is more likely to be relaxed, leading to more open communication.
- **E**ye contact: this is important to engage with the individual and make them feel that you are interested in them and that you are focused on your conversation with them.
- **T**ouch: this is an important non-verbal communication that can provide reassurance and comfort or demonstrate empathy when communicating with patients. However, be careful when using touch that it is appropriate to the person you are communicating with. Some people may feel awkward if a relative stranger physically touches them and we have to be aware of individual personal space and not invading this.
- **Y**our intuition: As discussed above, as you become more experienced you will develop intuitive understanding that will guide your actions.

2.3 Non-verbal communication

As demonstrated in *Section 2.1.3*, non-verbal communication is as important as verbal communication. Egan (2002) described the SOLER stance as a useful approach when thinking about non-verbal communication and, in particular, it can aid active listening:

- **S**it squarely in relation to the client
- **O**pen posture
- **L**ean slightly forward
- **E**ye – use and maintain appropriate eye contact
- **R**elaxed – try to look relaxed.

You will observe other interactions between the patient and perhaps family members or other care staff. It is important to be aware that not all communication is positive and in some instances, observed communication might require you to report a safeguarding concern.

2.4 Negative communication and malignant social psychology

Communication can be damaging as well as positive, and poor communication can damage self-esteem. Kitwood (1993) explores ways that communication and environment can contribute to the negative experiences of people who have dementia. Communication with other service user groups is equally important, to ensure that they are not disempowered. Negative regard for individuals can reinforce feelings of negative self-esteem and thus the way that practitioners communicate is important for wellbeing and person-centred care (*Table 2.1*).

Table 2.1 *Summary of negative communications (Kitwood, 1993)*

Treachery – using forms of deception in order to distract or manipulate
Disempowerment – not allowing the person to use the abilities that they do have
Infantilisation – treating a person in a patronising way
Intimidation – inducing fear through use of threats or physical power
Labelling – using a category such as dementia as the main basis for interacting with someone or explaining their behaviour
Stigmatisation – treating someone as a diseased object or outcast
Outpacing – providing information, presenting choices, etc. at a rate too fast for the person to understand; putting them under pressure to do things more rapidly than they can manage
Invalidation – failing to acknowledge the subjective reality of someone's experience
Banishment – sending a person away or excluding them (psychologically or physically)
Objectification – treating a person as if they were an object with no feelings
Ignoring – disregarding what somebody is saying or doing
Imposition – forcing a person to do something or denying them the possibility of choice
Withholding – refusing to give attention or meet an evident need
Accusation – blaming a person for actions or failures of action that arise from lack of ability to understand
Disruption – intruding suddenly or disturbingly upon a person's action or reflection
Mockery – making fun of a person's strange actions or remarks
Disparagement – telling a person that s/he is incompetent, useless, worthless, etc.; giving messages that are damaging to self-esteem

2.5 Positive communication

Kitwood (1993) also identified a number of ways of communicating positively with people with dementia. In the same way as malignant social psychology can be applied to other service user groups, we can use Kitwood's positive communication concepts to explore effective communication more generally. Many of these are principles of good practice in the provision of person-centred care that acknowledge the person as a unique individual with a unique set of experiences and skills. These are summarised in *Table 2.2*.

Table 2.2 *Summary of positive ways of communicating*

Recognition – acknowledging someone as a unique individual

Negotiation – consulting about preferences and needs

Collaboration – working on a shared task, using a person's abilities and strengths

Play – taking opportunities for spontaneity and self-expression

Celebration – sharing joyful experiences

Timalation – sharing sensuous or sensual experiences

Relaxation – resting either alone or with others

Validation – accepting the reality and power of someone's experience

Holding – providing a safe psychological space where vulnerabilities can be expressed

Facilitation – enabling a person to do what they would not otherwise be able to do

Creation – creating or offering opportunities for people to offer something to a social setting

Giving – enabling a person to give to others

ACTIVITY 2.3

Reflect on a recent practice encounter with a service user. Can you identify elements of negative and positive ways of communicating with this person? Reflect on how this knowledge will affect your future practice.

2.6 Tools for communication

There are various tools that nurses can use to help people to communicate.

2.6.1 Sign language

Sign language is a visual means of communicating using gestures, facial expression and body language. Sign language is used mainly by people who are deaf or have hearing impairments.

In Britain, the most common form of sign language is called British Sign Language (BSL). BSL has its own grammatical structure and syntax; as a language it is not dependent on, nor is it strongly related to spoken English. BSL was the preferred language of around 145,000 people within the UK in 2011.

For information on BSL and courses that you can undertake see www.british-sign.
co.uk/what-is-british-sign-language/

2.6.2 Picture boards

Picture boards are a type of communication board for individuals who are unable
to communicate using their voice. They may help individuals to communicate their
wants and needs while in hospital. They can be made up of simple pictures that an
individual can point to, or words/letters to spell out their needs.

2.6.3 Imagery

Following the death of Peter Connelly (Baby P) in 2007, Eileen Munro was
commissioned to write a report into children's safeguarding. One of the
recommendations of the report was that it is important to hear the views of children
and to hear their story where abuse or risk is identified. One way of hearing these
views, particularly where the child is very young or has communication difficulties,
is to use the 'Three Houses Model' (*Figure 2.2*). Practitioners can use this model to
help the child to verbalise what they like, what they are worried about and what they
would like to happen. The three houses template enables social workers to discuss a
child's likes/hobbies/strengths/protective factors, dislikes/worries and risks related to
the child and dreams/hopes/wishes. A health practitioner or social worker can either
ask a child to draw/write things for each house or assist them in doing so.

When communicating with service users it is also important to remember that more
than one communication form might help them to understand the information
better. For example, it may be useful to provide written information to supplement
verbal information that the person can refer back to.

ACTIVITY 2.4

In relation to the case study about Frank and Lizzie, consider the following conversation
between Lizzie and her daughter after a hospital visit.

Lucy (daughter): So when does Dad have his stitches out?

Lizzie: I think the doctor said that we have to go back and see him next month.

Lucy: That seems a long time. Did they give you an appointment?

Lizzie: No. They said we need to see the GP.

Lucy: Did they tell you how soon you need to see the GP? Do you think the GP might take
the stitches out?

Lizzie: I don't know. I tried to write it down but I was confused about what we had to do.

What could have helped Lizzie to understand the communication more effectively?

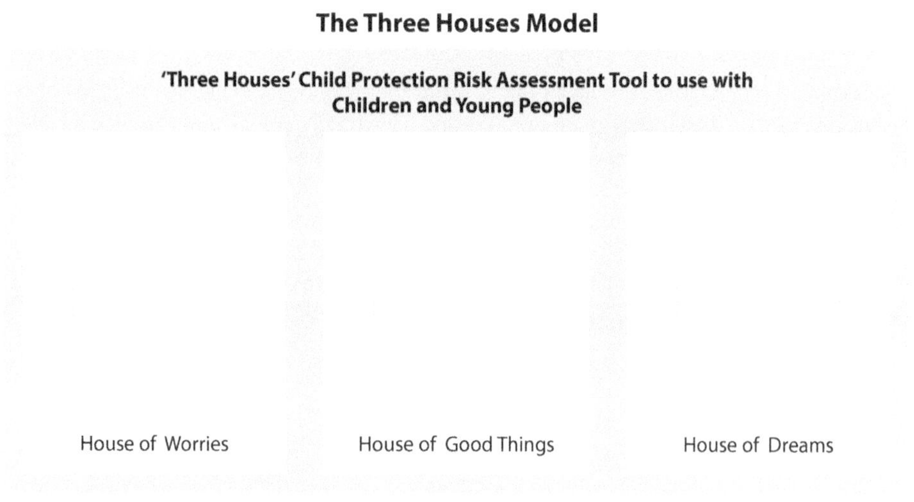

The Three Houses Model

'Three Houses' Child Protection Risk Assessment Tool to use with Children and Young People

House of Worries   House of Good Things   House of Dreams

Figure 2.2 *A typical 'Three Houses' template.*

2.7 The role of technology in nurse–patient communication

The role of technology for communicating with patients is multifaceted. It can be a tool for enhancing communication, for example to give information in a timely manner in a way that patients can refer back to. For example, clinical information could be given in a text version on a mobile device, allowing the user to have accurate written information on a device that enables them to read in a font of their choosing or have the message verbalised for them whenever they need it.

Health informatics aim to facilitate convenient and personalised care in primary and community care to empower patients and nurses to work as partners in care. Nurses need to embrace the use of digital technology such as E-obs (e.g. CareFlow Vitals, formerly known as VitalPAC) and electronic medicine prescriptions, engage with tablets and other portable devices, webcams and video conferencing as part of the nursing role.

There are, however, two key caveats when considering the use of technology in our communications. First, the level of digital literacy may differ between carers and service users, and assumptions about people's ability to use technology effectively should be avoided. We will consider the concept of 'digital exclusion' in *Chapter 8*. Secondly, "Health IT is about quality, safety and innovation – it is not an end in itself. Its development and use must always be patient centred, clinically owned and led, and aligned with local systems and aspirations" (Moore, 2009).

CHAPTER SUMMARY

This chapter has explored the skills needed for both verbal and non-verbal effective communication. The models for communicating have been outlined and good practice identified. The issues around poor communication and negative or malignant communication have also been discussed. Alternative ways of communicating such as using letter boards or interpreters have been included as areas for consideration in practice. Clinical examples include communicating with children or older adults who have some degree of cognitive impairment. In the final section, the relevance of technology and health informatics for organisational communication has been reviewed.

Reflection

Identify at least three things that you have learned from this chapter.	1. .... 2. .... 3. ....
How do you plan to use this knowledge within clinical practice?	1. .... 2. .... 3. ....
How will you evaluate the effectiveness of your plan?	1. .... 2. .... 3. ....
What further knowledge and evidence do you need?	1. .... 2. .... 3. ....

FURTHER READING

Age UK (2019) Safeguarding older people from abuse and neglect. Factsheet 78, January 2019. Available from: www.ageuk.org.uk/globalassets/age-uk/documents/factsheets/fs78_safeguarding_older_people_from_abuse_fcs.pdf

This factsheet explains the law on safeguarding adults to help you decide what to do if you think an older person is being abused or neglected, or may be at risk of abuse or neglect. Whether you know the person through your role as a professional, carer, relative, neighbour or friend, you have an important part to play in helping to safeguard them. Safeguarding means protecting people's right to live in safety, free from abuse and neglect. Any form of abuse or neglect is unacceptable, no matter what justification or reason may be given for it. It is very important that older people are aware of this and they know support is available. (Note that this factsheet describes the situation in England; there are differences in legislation and procedures in Northern Ireland, Scotland and Wales.)

Pavord, E. & Donnelly, E. (2015) *Communication and Interpersonal Skills*. Banbury: Lantern Publishing.

This second edition enables nursing and healthcare students to improve their communication and interpersonal skills. It provides an introduction to the theory that underpins communication studies and offers opportunities for students to reflect on their own practice. The book gives students helpful guidelines and tips, while emphasising that successful communication depends on the quality of the relationship.

Egan, G. (2002) *The Skilled Helper: a problem-management and opportunity-development approach to helping*, 7th edition. Pacific Grove, CA: Brooks/Cole.

This seminal text, now in its 7th edition, uses true-life examples and a three-stage model to explain 'helping' others. It focuses on skills for improving understanding and enabling change.

RCN guidelines on communication methods – useful professional guidance that looks at five important aspects of communication (see www.rcni.com/hosted-content/rcn/first-steps/communication-methods).

Chapter 3
Decision-making in the ASPIRE process

LEARNING OUTCOMES

This chapter covers the following key issues:

- Decision-making – definition and theory

- Problem-solving

- Critical thinking

- Ethical decision-making

- Mental capacity considerations

- Decision-making tools and frameworks.

By the end of this chapter, you should be able to:

- understand how decision-making underpins the care process

- identify and use appropriately the different types of decision-making tools

- understand how to involve your patients and their families and carers in the decision-making process

- make effective decisions and contribute to collaborative decision-making.

While many elements of the NMC platforms which make up the standards of proficiency for registered nurses are covered, this chapter has particular reference to (NMC, 2018b):

- Platform 3: Assessing needs and planning care

For further detailed mapping please see *Appendix 1* – Detailed mapping to *Future Nurse: standards of proficiency for registered nurses*.

3.1 Introduction

Care planning is based on a process of decision-making and integral to this is the ability to solve problems within the care situation. There are many theoretical approaches to problem-solving and decision-making but all come with the caveat that both problems and their solutions involve a myriad of variables and the outcome can be dependent on an individual care recipient's personal choice, one they may be reluctant to share with the care-giver.

Decision-making is a complex cognitive process often defined by choosing a particular course of action from alternatives following deliberation or judgement.

3.1.1 Types of decision

A decision is a type of judgement and there are different types of decisions. Some decisions might be based on a physical need, such as buying food; other decisions could be a response to an emotional need, for example buying a gift for someone.

Clinical decision-making ranges from the simple to the very complex. Most organisations try to support effective decision-making by providing pathways or protocols for staff to follow. For example, if a patient has a cardiac arrest, the responding crash team will follow the current national guidelines and algorithms. This ensures that all patients have treatment that is based on best evidence to give the best clinical outcome.

Clinical decisions can be:
- Routine – these usually do not cause difficulty or disagreement, for example collecting a urine sample if an infection is suspected.
- Urgent – these have an immediate response, such as the decision to commence CPR.
- Considered – these require input from a number of different people, each of whom may be affected by the decision made and who have the expectation if not the right to be involved. Think about complex discharge plans for patients returning home.

3.2 Decision-making models and tools

There are a number of theoretical models and tools that attempt to support effective decision-making, and we consider some of them in this section.

3.2.1 Decision-making models

One model to improve decision-making is the managerially-based model proposed by Marquis and Huston (2008, p. 26), which has the following stages:
1. Set objectives
2. Search for alternatives
3. Evaluate alternatives
4. Choose

5. Implement
6. Follow up and control

In this model the decision is made at step 4, but many decision-making models have similarities. Another popular decision-making model is the DECIDE framework. The DECIDE model is the acronym of six particular activities needed in the decision-making process (Guo, 2008):

- D = define the problem
- E = establish the criteria
- C = consider all the alternatives
- I = identify the best alternative
- D = develop and implement a plan of action
- E = evaluate and monitor the solution and feedback when necessary.

ACTIVITY 3.1

Stacey is 37 and has a learning disability. You notice that she is going to the toilet to pass urine frequently and seems uncomfortable and more quiet than usual. Use the DECIDE framework to aid your decisions:

- What is the problem? (Ask Stacey to say what she thinks the issue is.)
- What data would you want to consider (e.g. urine sample, check temperature)?
- How might you approach resolving the problem?
- Which of the options available would be the best first option? Has Stacey had a urine infection previously? How was it resolved?
- Do you think Stacey might need antibiotic therapy?
- How would you implement the action plan?
- How would you evaluate the outcome?

Now consider the same situation about Stacey and apply the Marquis and Huston model described above. Do you have an opinion about which model is easier to use?

There are some common problems with these models:

- It can take time to implement them fully.
- Individuals may try to make decisions without being completely clear about the goals or aim of the decision.
- The care interventions can fail because decisions were made using limited available knowledge and information. The care-giver and care recipient should have complete and accurate information to ensure the best outcome, although it is worth acknowledging that often a decision has to be made where information is not complete or fully accurate.
- Problem-solvers may be limited in their generation of alternative solutions, so the generation of choices is important. It is also important to think logically during the process.
- There is a risk of generalising and assuming consequence (without evidence).
- It can also be difficult sometimes to make a choice and act decisively.
  A consequence of recognising many alternatives is that the decision-making may be paralysed by choice.

3.2.2 Decision-making tools

One tool is a **decision grid**, which allows the visual comparison of a number of alternatives against any criteria (*Table 3.1*). The criteria can be anything of relevance, e.g. the cost of an intervention, carer preferences or workforce availability.

ACTIVITY 3.2: FRANK AND LIZZIE

Thinking about Frank and Lizzie, they have been invited to their local Salvation Army annual event, which includes having a meal with friends and enjoying social contact. They have missed having contact with the social group and both would like to attend; however, the decision to go is multifaceted. There would be positive aspects in going to the event but also some considerations.

Use the decision grid example shown in *Table 3.1* and suggest further criteria that you might consider.

Table 3.1 *Example of a decision grid*

	Criterion 1	Criterion 2	Criterion 3	Criterion 4
	Enabling Frank and Lizzie to remain connected to their social life as their increasing social isolation is worsening their mental health	The need to keep Frank and Lizzie safe, so physical considerations of transport and the accommodation at the event, e.g. availability of lifts	Lizzie and Frank's sense of autonomy and control	Their ability to cope with their physical challenges, e.g. eating in public
Option 1 – decline the invitation	May compound their isolation as Frank and Lizzie feel disappointed that they are missing out	No obvious issue but any social contact can alert others to declines in health or wellbeing	May protect the couple from any embarrassment or worry about how they will cope	No challenge to overcome

(continued)

Table 3.1 *(continued)*

Option 2 – either Frank or Lizzie attend alone	Either party may feel isolated or unsure by being separated and worry for one another during the separation	Transport and assessment of the physical environment is required	If the decision is for one of the couple to attend and represent them both, then the sense of autonomy and control may be achieved	May determine which one of the couple decides to attend
Option 3 – accept but attend for a limited time only	Enables social contact	Need to ensure transport, etc. is available	Again, if the decision is led by the couple this may be a good option	May give the ability to avoid the need to eat in public or use the toilet, etc.
Alternative 3 – accept and stay for the whole event	Helps to reduce social isolation	Consideration must be made to this	Ditto!	Reassurance and consideration must be given to how the couple can be helped to address any physical issues such as availability of an accessible toilet and food that Frank is able to manage

Another tool is the **decision tree**, which demonstrates the decision-making process by illustrating the possible decisions and outcomes of those decisions (Wu *et al.*, 2005). Essentially it allows visualisation of different outcomes and enables the processing of information by trying to illustrate the logical development of a decision and its alternatives and outcomes. To be able to successfully use decision trees, the user must have sufficient knowledge to identify alternative decisions and the different outcomes and probabilities related to these decisions.

We can use a decision tree in relation to Stacey's situation in *Activity 3.1*, as shown in *Figure 3.1*:

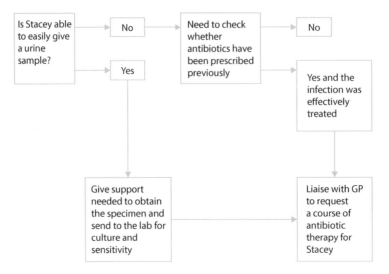

Figure 3.1 *Example of a decision tree.*

ACTIVITY 3.3

Look at the decision tree. Consider what decisions may be added. For example, you might consider the clinical value of waiting before using antibiotic therapy.

With any approach it is worth asking some key questions:

- Are the objectives clear?
- Is it patient-focused or organisation-focused?
- Is the evidence accurate?
- When was the assessment carried out and by whom?
- Does the decision-maker have the skills to make the decision?
- Was the assessor the right person… what is their bias?
- Have the alternatives been fully explored?
- Did you ask the patient/can you ask the patient? Is the logic sound?
- Are all parties considered? (Parties will include the patient, family, other professionals, the organisation [legal point of view].)

3.3 **Complex decisions**

In a healthcare setting, it is likely that a clinical decision will be complicated due to the nature of issues involved. Complex decisions usually have elements of:

- uncertainty
- intricacy
- risk
- alternatives
- personal impacts.

3.3.1 Uncertainty

For every decision we make, it is certain that some level of uncertainty will exist. There are things that we know, things that we don't know, things that we know we don't know, and things that we don't know that we don't know. That is to say, we can never be 100% certain of anything. The more uncertainty that exists with making a decision, the more complex it becomes.

3.3.2 Intricacy

The more interrelated factors involved in a decision, the more complex it becomes. If a decision leads to another difficult decision, then the original decision must have been a complex one (at least it should have been considered one). There is evidence available to show that nurses would rather use information gained verbally from people than research evidence (Thompson and Dowding, 2009). Why do you think that is the case?

3.3.3 Risk

Every decision has a certain level of risk (possibility of a negative outcome) associated with it. Some things, such as accepting a new job offer, may have a relatively low risk of negative consequences. Others, such as trying to drive a seriously injured accident victim to a hospital 20 miles away, have a relatively high risk of negative consequences associated with them. The more risk a decision has, the more complex it is.

3.3.4 Alternatives

For every decision, there is an alternative choice that can be made. Sometimes the only alternative is to do nothing, but this is rarely the case. The more alternative choices available to you, and thus alternative outcomes, the more complex the decision may be.

3.3.5 Personal impacts

For every decision, there may be personal considerations that may cloud or bias the judgement of the decision-maker, leading to subjective rather than objective outcomes. Examples include personal experiences such as family members being treated for cancer; and bias based on how we place value on health challenges, such as bias against smokers or individuals whose health issues are related to obesity or risk-taking behaviours.

3.4 Considerations for making good decisions

There are a number of critical elements in decision-making that should always be considered:

- It is essential that decisions have a clear objective or aim(s).
- Decisions are based on knowledge and so the acquisition of knowledge and information is a clear and important need (for both care professionals and clients).

- As problem-solvers gather information it must be recognised that preference is not mistaken for fact. This is why it is so important that many alternatives are generated in the decision-making process.

Several factors need to be considered to support these elements.

3.4.1 The individual

Individual decisions are based on the individual value system regardless of how objective the criteria – value judgements will always play a part (Marquis and Huston, 2008). Value judgements can be referred to as intuition based on past experiences and professionalism, but it is essential to think carefully about the decisions made and justify them according to objective criteria. Developing self-awareness and reflective practice is an important element in problem-solving outcomes. We all have a cultural lens through which we view the world and it is easy to assume that patients will share our personal beliefs and values, but this needs to be checked – it is not enough to say that the intention was good.

Individuals will differ in terms of:
- personal values and beliefs – the ethical perspective (Seedhouse, 2009)
- life experiences and professional experience – novice to expert practitioner (Benner, 1984)
- willingness to take risks as against adherence to protocol (Dimond, 2005)
- ways of thinking – logical, worst case scenario
- influences of NMC or employer.

There are a number of characteristics that successful decision-makers demonstrate, such as:
- willingness to make decisions
- ability to make sound decisions
- characteristics of effective leadership (Covey, 1989)
- courageous
- creative and energetic.

There are also different types of decision-making styles:
- decisive – depends on less data to arrive at one decision
- integrative – uses all available data and identifies multiple alternatives
- hierarchic – focuses on a large amount of information but arrives at one alternative or solution
- flexible – uses a small amount of data while generating multiple alternatives and may change as information is reinterpreted.

3.4.2 Collaborative decision-making

THE USE OF COLLABORATION – AN EXAMPLE

You are in the basement of a building and there are three light switches.

You are told that there are three bulbs, one on each floor (ground floor, first floor and second floor).

You need to find out which light switch connects to which bulb. The bulbs are not visible to you until you go onto each floor.

You can only go upstairs once.

How will you determine which switch is responsible for which bulb?

Try to find the answer by yourself, then try asking other people to help you figure it out. There is an answer (see *Appendix 2*)!

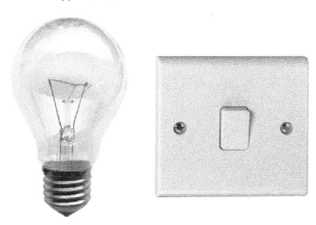

How is this relevant to clinical decision-making? Sometimes the best decisions will emerge from a group of people sharing ideas and thoughts. The aim of multidisciplinary team members is to try to see the patient's needs from a range of different perspectives so that often creative responses can be taken into account.

Considered decisions within a care situation will normally entail shared or collaborative decision-making and there are a number of steps that must be considered when working in this way. It is essential to consider the context of the service user/client and the context of the healthcare practitioner, the context of the main care-giver (if appropriate) and the context of the situation (Dalton & Gottlieb, 2003). This will be enabled if the following steps are taken:
1. Develop a partnership.
2. Review the service user's preferences for information.
3. Establish the service user's preferences for role in decision-making.
4. Ascertain the service user's ideas.
5. Identify choices.

6. Present evidence.
7. Negotiate a decision.
8. Agree an action plan.

3.4.3 Involving the patient and carer

Patient and carer involvement in health and social care is a fundamental policy imperative. However, there are a number of different ways that users and carers can be involved in the decision-making processes in health and social care, involving different levels of partnership and empowerment. There are variations in the nature of collaborative working between different geographical localities and different service user and carer groups, and user and carer involvement in decision-making may be seen as tokenistic. Arnstein's 'ladder of citizenship participation (see *Figure 3.2*) is useful to illustrate this, identifying different ways of engaging users and carers and the degree to which this involves and empowers them (Arnstein, 1969).

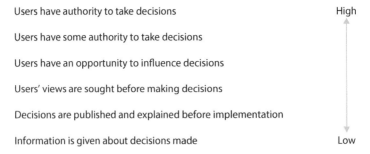

Users have authority to take decisions   High

Users have some authority to take decisions

Users have an opportunity to influence decisions

Users' views are sought before making decisions

Decisions are published and explained before implementation

Information is given about decisions made   Low

Figure 3.2 *Levels of empowerment (Braye and Preston-Shoot, 1995).*

Table 3.2 gives some examples of how patients may be involved in the decision-making process in health and social care.

Table 3.2 *Levels and methods of patient involvement (Oliviere* et al., *1998)*

Level of involvement	Methods	Tasks
Informed	Newsletters, leaflets, posters, radio	Informing service users about entitlements, resources, new services
Consultation	Focus or discussion groups, semi-structured interviews, questionnaires	Finding out views on services
Collaboration/ partnership	Committees, working groups	Agreeing priorities for service improvements
User control	Self-help and support groups, user groups	Users decide priorities and action in response to need

3.4.4 Information

Having the right information and getting it to the right people at the right time – in a form they can understand, engage with and contribute to – will help individuals take control of their own care, improving self-management, shared decision-making and more informed choices (Department of Health, 2012b). If we are bombarded with information how do we filter the information? The Royal College of Nursing (2011) suggests nurses should be competent in:

- identifying **why** information is needed
- identifying **what** information is required
- carrying out a **search** to find information
- **evaluating** how the information meets the identified need
- **using information** and knowledge inclusively, legally and ethically
- **managing** information
- **creating** new information or knowledge.

With all of this information around us evidence shows that we often have to make quick decisions where we have "irreducible uncertainty" (Thompson and Dowding, 2009). In other words, we make decisions where we do not have all the information at hand.

The Royal College of Nursing states: "As well as timely alerts, Information Communication Technology (ICT) can provide sophisticated decision support...." (Royal College of Nursing, 2012). However, there are dangers in incorporating electronic information in decision-making activities, such as reliance on technology over your clinical competence and awareness. It could lead to forgetting the human being receiving care.

There is a wide range of information sources available in health and social care. For example:

- Medical/nursing notes
- Verbally from patients or relatives
- Policies and procedures
- Lab reports
- From machines – Dinamaps/CareFlow Vitals, formerly known as VitalPAC (National Institute for Health and Care Excellence, 2016)
- X-rays and scans
- Handover
- Own memory and experience
- Instinct
- Colleagues
- NMC
- Journals
- Books
- The internet
- Telephone
- Social media
- Union

Can you add to the list of 'sources of information' above? How would you ensure 'legitimacy' or evidence-based decision-making when considering, for example, whether to use the internet as a source, or patient-reported information or even your own instinct?

3.4.5 Critical thinking

It is important to think critically when making clinical decisions (Gambrill, 2012). Critical thinking is reasoning in a manner that generates and examines questions and problems. Intuition and feelings are considered as an individual weighs, clarifies and evaluates evidence, arguments and conclusions (Stark, 1995).

Critical thinking skills include knowledge, experience, judgement and evaluation as well as interpretation of context. The decision-maker will engage in affective listening and application of moral reasoning and values. A disposition to critical thinking includes a number of traits (Shin *et al.*, 2006):
- Open-mindedness
- Inquisitiveness
- Truth seeking
- Analyticity
- Systematicity
- Self-confidence
- Maturity of judgement.

When thinking about theoretical models, an assumption might be that all decision-making is carefully considered.
- Could the idea that decisions are a cognitive process be challenged?
- Do you think that some decisions are intuitive?
- Have you heard nurses saying that they had a 'gut feeling'?
- What do you think this means for evidence-based practice?

A definition of nursing intuition could be: "A process whereby the nurse knows something about a patient that cannot be verbalized, that is verbalized with difficulty or for which the source of knowledge cannot be determined" (Young, 1987).

3.4.6 Clinical judgement

Clinical judgement is defined as the "assessment of alternatives" (Thompson and Dowding, 2009). Experience and expertise affect the way in which nurses make decisions (Standing, 2017). When making decisions nurses must consider the following strategies:
- Look for what does not fit rather than what does (confirmation bias).
- Be specific when estimating probabilities, such as risk of falls.
- Consider reasons why a judgement may be incorrect.

- Respect ambiguity in information by remaining open.
- Think about the context and possible defensive practices.

Frank is not eating very much and seems 'off colour' so Lizzie has made an appointment with you as the Nursing Associate in the GP practice. You have recorded Frank's vital signs and his temperature is slightly raised but it is a warm afternoon. He says he feels 'okay' and his other observations are within the normal parameters. Lizzie feels sure that Frank is 'brewing something' but can't be more specific.

What are your considerations?

What advice would you give to Frank and Lizzie?

How much value do you give to Lizzie's concerns?

Points to consider
- Check urine sample – may be developing a urine infection.
- Ask about breathing – does Frank have a cough or 'flu-like' symptoms (early signs of upper respiratory chest infection)
- Ask about bowel movements – constipation can impact on wellbeing.
- How is Frank's emotional health – is he stressed or more anxious than usual?
- Is Frank taking his medication or has he made any changes to his medication practices, such as herbal remedies?
- Check blood sugar – may be lower or higher than usual and need further investigation.

How do you respond when you cannot determine any health issues that could answer Lizzie's concerns?

3.4.7 Ethical considerations

Decision-making must reflect the four ethical principles (*Figure 3.3*).

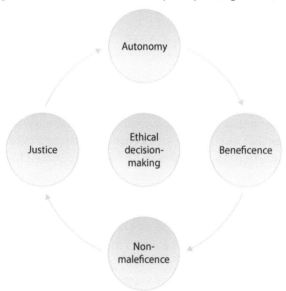

Figure 3.3 *Dimensions of ethical decision-making.*

Autonomy – the right of a person to make their own decisions and direct their life; think about Stacey and her possible reluctance to provide a urine sample. Even though we might think that this is an unwise decision, if Stacey has mental capacity (see *Section 3.4.8*), she has the right to make autonomous decisions.

Beneficence – the responsibility of doing good and so providing benefit or beneficial treatment/care to the person; consider the use of covert medicine administration to patients who have cognitive impairment.

Non-maleficence – the responsibility of avoiding harm to the person. Under the law, decisions can be made about the care of someone who lacks the capacity to make a decision themselves if it is deemed to be in the best interests of that individual. This is known as a deprivation of liberty standard (for further information, see Law Society, 2015).

Justice – the responsibility to be equitable and fair in the way we treat others. Think about non-judgemental care and preferential treatment for 'favourite patients'. It is human nature to like some people more than others, but as a nurse we have a duty to be non-judgemental. Consider the following scenario:

CASE STUDY 3.1

You are working in an orthopaedic ward and two male patients have been admitted. John is a 17-year-old who was the driver of a car involved in a road traffic collision in which he sustained a fractured femur and concussion. George is a 42-year-old man who had met his 14-year-old daughter after she had attended a party at a friend's house so that he could walk her home safely. John was high on drugs and had stolen a car, which he was driving recklessly. He was speeding and ignored a red light, hitting George and his daughter as they crossed the road. George sustained multiple injuries and his daughter was pronounced dead at the scene of the accident. Although you may have views about John and his behaviour, you have a duty to treat him and care for him in a fair and just way.

When making decisions in the caring relationship, consideration must therefore be given to:

- The importance of duty or rights in the decision-making process – for example whether practitioners in healthcare have a moral obligation to act in a certain way.
- Although we may not think a service user is making the decision that we would, people have the right to make their own decisions. Under the Mental Capacity Act (Department of Health, 2005), people who are deemed to have mental capacity have the right to make unwise decisions about their future.
- Whether there are any absolute or fixed principles that guide behaviour, these could be as ethical principles such as 'above all do no harm' but can also be seen in professional codes such as the Nursing and Midwifery Council Code (2018a). New data protection laws govern what information is kept and how any information is used. It would be worth checking your organisation's patient record policies for guidance.
- The principle of universalism and consistency in decision-making, which can be argued to reflect the principle of utility – the need to achieve the greatest

good for the greatest number – and also the principle of justice, which is about equity and could relate to issues such as distribution of services and resources. A principle of the NHS Constitution (NHS England, 2015) states that decisions should be based on individual clinical need.

- The issues of dignity and worth, welfare or wellbeing and social justice are important (Banks, 2006). All care should be anti-discriminatory, regardless of whether the patient is a prisoner, drug user or discourteous to staff.

3.4.8 Mental capacity

It is also very important to consider the five principles of the Mental Capacity Act:

1. A person must be assumed to have capacity unless it is established that they lack capacity.
2. A person is not to be treated as unable to make a decision unless all practicable steps to help them to do so have been taken without success.
3. A person is not to be treated as unable to make a decision merely because they make an unwise decision.
4. Any action or decision made on behalf of a person who lacks capacity must be done, or made, in their best interests.
5. Before any action or decision is made, it should be achieved in a way that is less restrictive of the person's rights and freedom of action.

ACTIVITY 3.7: FRANK AND LIZZIE

Frank has lost weight and is not enjoying eating food. He is uncomfortable when eating due to his new dentures and has lost interest in food. He has stated that he will only eat tinned soup twice a day and will refuse any other food. Lizzie is worried about his weight loss.

Thinking about the mental capacity principles, use a decision tree or a decision grid to explore the outcomes and, referring to the ethical framework above, try to decide what you should do.

Sometimes it is necessary for decisions to be made on behalf of people who lack the capacity to make those decisions themselves. This can be planned in advance through the use of a Lasting Power of Attorney, where a person can be nominated in advance to make decisions on behalf of the patient if they become unable to make those decisions for themselves. This can take two forms:

1. Lasting Power of Attorney for financial decisions.
2. Lasting Power of Attorney for health and welfare decisions.

FRANK AND LIZZIE

As their health deteriorates they have filled out the paperwork to authorise their son and eldest daughter to make decisions on their behalf. They decided to ask their son as their eldest child, and their eldest daughter as she is the one who sees the most of them. This planned approach has given Frank and Lizzie the opportunity to discuss their preferences with their closest next of kin, so that they can make decisions that are in their best interests as well as respecting their wishes.

3.4.9 Environment

The impact that environment has on a decision is often underestimated.

Thinking back to the case study of Frank and Lizzie, can you identify physical and social factors that might affect their decision-making (e.g. the desire to stay in their own home)?

Human factors

Sometimes the broader environment of the work system design does not allow the most appropriate decisions to be made. The system is not designed with human interaction fully considered. For example, have you ever walked towards a door that had a handle but a sign saying 'push'? The message can be misleading: do you push the handle or pull it to open the door?

This is the basis of human factor science. Watch the short video at www.youtube.com/watch?v=aGZz3w5Hy8Y, which is a good introduction to what human factors means. It describes how it is important to make it easier for care staff to make safe decisions. A simplistic example is one in the world of health promotion. People often get 'peckish' during the working day. What would you do if the only access in your place of work to a snack was a vending machine full of chocolate and the alternative is a 15-minute walk to a shop where you can purchase fruit or other healthy choices? Employers may consider giving free fruit or using vending machines that have healthy snacks that make that choice accessible.

3.5 Model for effective decision-making

Good professional nursing practice rests on the ability to make sound professional judgements based upon clinical indicators. Effective decision-making is seen as the cornerstone of professional nursing practice, and is therefore the principle criterion by which clinical expertise is measured. Finally, it is important not to see decision-making as an isolated step in the ASPIRE process. It is everywhere in the process and this overview helps to demonstrate a model of decision-making which is present at every stage of the process. You DECIDE to take this approach and it informs the clinical and care decisions that you make:

- Use the 'Hello my name is….' introduction to the patient, and family if they are present. This allows the patient to give an implied consent to you speaking with them by returning the greeting.
- By stating clearly why you are speaking to the patient, you give the patient the opportunity to ask questions. It is essential to have the patient's involvement in any aspect of care. Listen attentively to their story.
- If you are requesting any information from the patient, you should explain why you need the information and what you will do with it. This is part of your responsibility to explain how you are protecting the patient information in line with General Data Protection Regulation (GDPR). You could also explain how confidentiality will be maintained.

- Ask for the patient's ideas, concerns and expectations so that you can address these issues in the care plan. It is important to ask about the patient's perception of their health and if appropriate, ask the relative as well. This should help your understanding about the level of independence/dependence that the patient has in meeting their own needs, as well as family involvement in care.
- It may be appropriate to use assessment tools to gather empirical, physiological data, for example temperature, heart rate and blood pressure. Other assessment tools might include nutritional assessment tools such as Malnutrition Universal Screening Tool (MUST).
- At some point during assessment, holistic needs will be reviewed (physical, emotional, psychological, cultural and social dimensions).
- The cognitive ability of the patient and capacity for independence might require the use of a mental health assessment tool such as the Mini Mental State Examination (MMSE) or the Hospital Anxiety and Depression Score (HADS).
- Once this information is gathered, it might be worth checking this against other sources of information such as care records to see whether the patient has deteriorated since a previous admission.
- When you have a clearer assessment of holistic needs, you should involve the patient in setting realistic goals, which may be short-term and long-term goals for each identified need. The care plan (see *Chapter 5*) should reflect the patient's needs and use professional and organisational guidelines using current best evidence. It is common to include an integrated care approach where other agencies might be involved, such as Social Services. The care plan may include health promotion or patient awareness focus.
- The patient should be asked to evaluate care and say whether they feel closer to the goals that were set. Comprehensive evaluation should be recorded in line with organisational and NMC guidelines. It is important to remember that patients may have a change in health status – continuous monitoring is essential so that plans can be amended as needed.

CHAPTER SUMMARY

This chapter has explored the issues around decision-making that are relevant across the ASPIRE process. A definition for decision-making has been offered and different types of decisions distinguished. The chapter includes practical advice and has explored decision-making tools and techniques which may be applicable in different situations and contexts. For example, the decision-making grid and decision tree were applied to different clinical scenarios. The context for decision-making was reviewed and real-life issues such as personal influences, risk and uncertainty were highlighted.

It is unusual to make a sound decision unilaterally, or without input from other healthcare stakeholders so the integrated decision-making topic was explored. Ethical dimensions and reference to mental health capability are important aspects in working with patients and involving them in making decisions. The involvement of patients in their care is vital and this was included in the chapter with an exploration of different levels of involvement of patient and carers. As in *Liberating the NHS* (Department of Health, 2012c) 'no decision about me, without me' resonates throughout the chapter.

Reflection

Identify at least three things that you have learned from this chapter.

1. ....
....

2. ....
....

3. ....
....

How do you plan to use this knowledge within clinical practice?

1. ....
....

2. ....
....

3. ....
....

How will you evaluate the effectiveness of your plan?

1. ....
....

2. ....
....

3. ....
....

What further knowledge and evidence do you need?

1. ....
....

2. ....
....

3. ....
....

FURTHER READING

Gambrill, E. (2012) *Critical Thinking in Clinical Practice: improving the quality of judgments and decisions*, 3rd edition. Hoboken, NJ: John Wiley & Sons, Inc.

This text examines the knowledge and skills of critical thinking, evidence-based practice, problem-solving, judgement and decision-making. These are essential to effectively serve clients in all types of clinical practices. The book explores how to address the challenges such as biases in thinking, as well as the skills to make well-informed, ethical decisions. Grounded in the belief that clinical decision-making is a challenging process that can be improved by honing the skills integral to evidence-based practice, it explores common sources of error and provides psychologists, counsellors, social workers and allied health professionals practical guidance with decision aids and applications of critical thinking skills to clinical decision-making.

Peters, S. (2012) *The Chimp Paradox: the mind management programme for confidence, success and happiness*. London: Vermilion.

Steve Peters explains the nature of your mind, and identifies three parts of the mind – the 'computer', the 'human' and the 'chimp'. Each part has different characteristics; for example, the computer is logical, organised and can process information very efficiently. The human element is sensible, rational and can make logical decisions, while the chimp part is like a chimp. This part of the mind is impulsive, emotional and easily jumps to conclusions (often incorrectly). The premise of the book is to provide strategies for managing your chimp so that you are able to make more balanced decisions. This is an easy-to-read text that you can go back to.

Kahneman, D. (2012) *Thinking, Fast and Slow*. London: Penguin.

The premise of the book is that your brain has two systems, one being the ancient limbic system and the other the more developed neocortex. Both parts have an influence on the decisions we make – the limbic system is effective in impulsive and reactive decisions whereas the neocortex is more deliberate and considered. Kahneman discusses judgement and complex decision-making underpinned by psychological research.

Lehrer, J. (2009) *The Decisive Moment: how the brain makes up its mind*. Edinburgh: Canongate Books.

This book explores how we make decisions. It uses anecdotes and examples throughout and at times it is gripping. The concept of intuition is analysed and situations such as landing an aircraft or manning a wartime submarine are used to explain how people make decisions. This book is easy to read and Lehrer attempts to answer questions using a scientific approach.

Chapter 4
Assessment

LEARNING OUTCOMES

This chapter covers the following key issues:

- The purpose of assessment
- The nature of assessment relating to the different client groups, e.g. children and the elderly
- Tools for assessment
- Application of assessment approaches and tools as applied to the case of Frank and Lizzie.

By the end of this chapter, you should be able to:

- undertake effective, evidence-based assessment
- understand why and when to use different tools and approaches to assessment
- assess needs in the context of the service users' and carers' lives.

While many elements of the NMC platforms that make up the standards of proficiency for registered nurses are covered, this chapter has particular reference to (NMC, 2018b):

- Platform 2: Promoting health and preventing ill health
- Platform 3: Assessing needs and planning care

For further detailed mapping please see *Appendix 1* – Detailed mapping to *Future Nurse: standards of proficiency for registered nurses*.

4.1 **Introduction**

Assessment is the first stage in the cyclical process of ASPIRE (*Figure 4.1*).

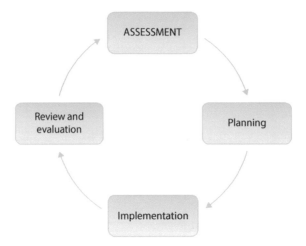

Figure 4.1 *The cyclical process of ASPIRE.*

Good assessment is fundamental to the cyclical process of care. If we fail to assess properly, there is a risk of interventions being based on guesswork or chance, or of a ritualised approach to the care process (Thompson and Thompson, 2008). Effective assessment is essential for the identification of problems as well as setting goals and planning interventions.

4.2 **Defining assessment**

Assessment is a holistic process that determines the planning and intervention stages of the care process. The assessment stage of care is sometimes referred to as being like having 'helicopter vision' (Thompson, 2005) as it provides an overview of the person in context. It is not simply about gathering information, determining a person's needs or deciding what services will best address their needs. A sound assessment is also fundamental for provision of high-quality care, as a narrow focus will limit the options for intervention, and inaccuracy will lead to inaccurate planning and interventions.

It is important, however, to distinguish between assessment and admission. There is overlap between the two, but the admission process does not provide a comprehensive assessment. Admission includes gathering initial information that might contribute towards the assessment, but it also includes documenting essential administrative details about the patient.

4.3 **Models of care and assessment**

Models of care guide practitioners in terms of what they should assess. There are various models in health and social care that place emphasis on different theoretical approaches and provide a framework to guide practice. For example, a number of different models for nursing have developed since the 1960s and 1970s, and these provide nurses with a mental picture to guide their practice.

4.3.1 Interaction models

Interaction models place the emphasis on the interaction between individuals and the way in which people behave on the basis of how they interpret a situation or interaction. Meanings and interpretations happen within a specific context and may be dependent on the individual's interactions with others. Interaction models have been used extensively in mental health nursing, with the emphasis on the importance of interactions between nurse and service user, and including concepts such as communication, role and self-concept.

Peplau's model is a good example of this type of model. For Peplau (1952), the focus of nursing was on the therapeutic interpersonal relationship between patient and nurse. Her model is based on humanistic theories and she emphasises the importance of two basic concepts – anxiety and communication, which she views as interrelated (Hayes & Llewellyn, 2008). If communication is seen as threatening in any way, then anxiety results, which is manifested either physically or psychologically. The role of the nurse in Peplau's model is thus tied up in the interpersonal process and the therapeutic relationship. Peplau sees the interpersonal process as having four sequential phases, which help individuals to problem-solve and emotionally mature. These phases are:

- orientation, where the nurse makes the care recipient aware of the availability of help
- identification, where the nurse facilitates the expression of feelings
- exploitation, where the nurse uses communication skills to help the care recipient view problems realistically, and work to reduce the anxiety so that they may personally grow
- resolution, the final phase, where the care recipient becomes independent and disengages from the interpersonal relationship.

ACTIVITY 4.1 – FRANK

Frank is admitted to A&E after falling and is in a distressed state.

Looking at the phases of Peplau's interpersonal process, give one or two examples of how the nurse caring for him can establish a therapeutic interpersonal relationship.

4.3.2 Developmental models

These models focus on stages or processes of development or change to explain the nurse/patient interaction. Self-care, activities of daily living and human needs models all have commonalities in their focus on the human need for life and health. One of the most widely used nursing models is the activities of living model devised by Roper *et al.* (2000), which identifies 12 activities that are required for living and health:

- Maintaining a safe environment
- Communicating
- Breathing

- Eating and drinking
- Eliminating
- Personal cleansing and dressing
- Controlling body temperature
- Mobilising
- Working and playing
- Expressing sexuality
- Sleeping
- Dying.

Dying is incorporated as an important aspect of human existence. This model guides nursing practitioners to important aspects of life and health, which can form a framework for assessment, although the practitioner may need to make a judgement about which parts of the model are relevant to each service user.

ACTIVITY 4.2 – FRANK

Think again about Frank after his admission to A&E. Can you use this model to assess his needs in relation to each of the activities of living? Give at least one for each activity.

4.3.3 Systems models

Systems models use the general theory of systems to describe the focus of the nursing situation. The service user is regarded as a system within the context of other systems, and thus the models focus on the way that the person interacts with stressors within these systems.

For example, the Roy Adaptation Model (Andrews and Roy, 2009) uses systems theory to explore how nurses can help service users to adapt to their stressors and their environment. This model comprises the four domain concepts of person, health, environment and nursing, and involves a six-step nursing process. The person is seen as an open, adaptive system. People use coping skills to deal with 'stressors' and health is seen as the process of being and becoming an integrated and whole person. The goal of nursing is, therefore, to promote adaptation in each of four modes – physiological, self-concept, role function and interdependence (social functioning) (Andrews and Roy, 2009).

Roy uses a six-step nursing process:
1. Assessment of behaviour in each of the four modes is assessed as adaptive or ineffective as compared to norms.
2. Assessment of stimuli or the factors that influence behaviour is undertaken.
3. Nursing diagnosis identifies the ineffective behaviours and probable cause.
4. Goal setting involves realistic and attainable goals set in collaboration with the person.
5. Intervention is where the stimuli are addressed, using strategies that are appropriate for the individual's adaptation.
6. Evaluation assesses the degree of change and ineffective behaviours are then reassessed and interventions revised.

4.3.4 Other approaches

Assessment of needs can adopt a **deficit approach** to care, identifying problems and solutions to address these problems. On the other hand, a **needs-led assessment** identifies problems in context and also identifies normal coping strategies and strengths, and can therefore maximise service user independence (Parry-Jones and Soulsby, 2001).

LIZZIE

Since fracturing her ankle recently, Lizzie has been having increasing mobility problems and has sustained minor injuries from a number of falls in the house and while going to the shops.

A deficit model of assessment might see the problem in terms of the mobility and assess Lizzie as needing to go into care to protect her from further risk.

A needs-led assessment would focus on Lizzie's needs and her perspective and her coping strategies. She may feel that she needs adaptations to the house and mobility aids to help her to get about more freely in order to help her to stay independent.

ACTIVITY 4.3 – FRANK

Think about Frank going to the hospital to see the specialist about his mouth ulcers. Can you identify Frank's needs from a problem-solving and a deficit perspective?

The **recovery model** that is used in mental health practice is a good example of a theoretical model that is person-centred and adopts a strengths approach to care management (Fawcett and Karban, 2005). Similarly, the theory behind the Single Assessment Process is that the service user and carer should be central to the needs assessment, so that their strengths and preferred ways of coping can be identified.

ACTIVITY 4.4 – FRANK

Thinking again about Frank, identify the strengths that he has and how his coping strategies can be utilised to manage his current difficulties.

Under the Care Act (2014), local authorities are required to use a strengths based approach to assessment, which focuses on what the individual can do and then identifies the support that might be available to them within the wider community.

Department of Health (2014a) Care Act. London: HMSO

4.4 How do we assess people's needs?

Now that we have looked at models of care and the theoretical underpinning of assessment, we can start to discuss how we go about assessing a person's needs in health and social care. Assessment involves a number of activities, including:

- identification of the problem or issue and sources of information
- collection and collation of relevant information

- assessing the information
- analysing and evaluating the information
- developing a plan of intervention.

In order to assess a patient's needs, we need to ask a number of questions:
- What is the purpose of the assessment?
- What types of information need to be collected and to whom are they relevant?
- Whose views should be incorporated?
- How do we make sense of the information to inform planning and intervention?
- How do we record the information?

4.5 The purpose of assessment

Assessments in health and social care can be undertaken for a number of different reasons including:
- providing a plan of care
- prevention of risk
- provision of advice and information to support independence and self-care.

Knowing where to begin can be difficult, but identification of purpose will help to provide you with guidance.

The Single Assessment Process (SAP), introduced as part of the *National Service Framework for Older People* (Department of Health, 2001b), is an example of a model for interdisciplinary assessment, which focuses on the needs of older adults. Using the Single Assessment Process as an example (see *Appendix 3*), we can see that there are different levels of assessment that may not all be carried out when the service user has initial contact with health and social care agencies. It may not be possible to assess all needs at once, and the assessment process may need to be staged. Within the Single Assessment Process there are four types of assessment:

1. **Contact assessment**: this type of assessment is concerned with identification of the:
   - nature of the presenting needs
   - significance of the need for the older person
   - length of time that the need has been experienced
   - potential solutions identified by the older person
   - recent life changes or events which are relevant to the current needs
   - perceptions of family members and carers.
2. **Overview assessment**: this type of assessment is carried out when a more rounded assessment is needed. Within this assessment, there are different domains:
   - user's perspective
   - clinical background (which often includes multi-pathology and normal senescence)

- disease prevention
- personal care and physical wellbeing
- senses
- mental health
- relationships
- safety
- immediate environment and resources.

3. **Specialist assessment**: this type of assessment is carried out when there is a need to explore specific needs in detail and is carried out by the most appropriate qualified person.

4. **Comprehensive assessment**: this is carried out when a specialist assessment indicates all or most of the domains of the SAP are involved, when the service user has a complex set of needs to be addressed. It involves a range of different professionals or teams, although a geriatrician often takes the lead role.

Contact assessment and overview assessment would usually be carried out early in the service user's engagement with health and social care services, so that immediate needs can be established, as well as the service user's and carer's own abilities and strategies to manage any problems or needs.

In some situations, a comprehensive holistic assessment is not appropriate. Consider working in an A&E department where a patient comes in in a collapsed state. The purpose of the initial assessment would be to establish immediate goals for intervention and would focus around airway, breathing and circulation (ABC) as life-saving interventions may be required (*Figure 4.2*). It may be that further assessment would need to take place once the initial crisis has been addressed.

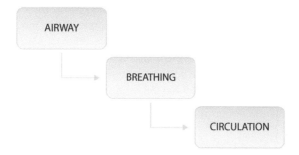

Figure 4.2 *The ABC framework in emergency care.*

LIZZIE

Lizzie's older sister, Mary, was visiting from Norfolk for a few days; they were enjoying some rare time together. Mary had recently been stressed because of some financial worries and wanted to confide in Lizzie. Lizzie and Mary decided to prepare and cook an evening meal and shared a taxi to the local supermarket. They were leaving the store with bags of fresh vegetables when Lizzie had a sudden pain across her back and felt very breathless. She collapsed to the floor and there were 'no signs of life' so Mary called 999 for an ambulance.

On arrival, the paramedic immediately looked inside Lizzie's mouth and used a head tilt, chin lift technique to ensure that Lizzie's tongue was not obstructing her **AIRWAY** and at the same time looked at Lizzie's chest to see if it was rising with an inhalation of breath to check for **BREATHING**. She had her ear close to Lizzie's mouth to try to feel for breath at the same time. The paramedic was counting for 10 seconds to see if there was any sign of life. She was also trying to see if she could feel a carotid pulse in Lizzie's neck to establish whether there was any **CIRCULATION**.

This was the initial assessment to establish the cause of Lizzie's collapse and the paramedic would also quickly try to establish whether she had any known cardiac problems.

ACTIVITY 4.5 – LIZZIE

Using the Roy Adaptation Model, assess Lizzie's needs when she collapsed and identify her needs in each of the four modes (physiological, self-concept, role function and interdependence).

Identify possible goals and how to evaluate them.

ACTIVITY 4.6 – FRANK

Consider the type of assessment needed for the following scenarios:
1. Frank has been referred by his dentist to attend the specialist at the hospital as he has some ulceration and sinister 'lumps' in his mouth. What information do you think would be essential for the specialist to understand?
2. Frank has become more forgetful and his GP has asked him to attend the memory clinic for assessment. How long do you think the assessment might take and where will the key information be obtained?

4.6 Assessment in context

From *Activity 4.6* it can be seen that the purpose of assessment very much depends upon the context and the immediate and longer-term needs of the person.

Thinking about Lizzie in the situation above, where she suddenly collapsed, we can see that there is a need to assess her vital signs to manage the immediate medical crisis. Once that is resolved, there may be a need to assess her other health problems. It is unlikely that her detached retina problem is significant in her collapse but at some point the paramedic will want to contact Frank or a member of her family, so that they know that she has collapsed and needs hospital assessment.

An assessment of an individual's needs has to be considered in relation to the psychosocial and environmental context of that person's life. People make sense of health and illness from their own subjective experiences, and so attitudes and beliefs regarding need and addressing need are shaped within the individual, family and community/cultural context (Kleinman, 1988). It is therefore important when working from a person-centred perspective to identify and understand the subjective experiences and understandings that the individuals have. It is also important to see beyond the need that is presented and identified, to understand how that need has arisen, how it impacts on the individual and the coping strategies that they already have that can be built upon.

4.7 Types of information to be collected

Assessment is essentially about the collection of data to produce a plan of care and intervention. Data can be derived from the primary sources (the person him/herself), secondary sources (practitioner's observations, data from family and friends), or tertiary sources (other health and social care providers, service user records).

Assessment, then, is an interpersonal activity, which involves a relationship between the practitioner and service user. The data collected may be either objective or subjective, and requires the practitioner to have a number of skills to assess the area or areas of concern (*Table 4.1*).

Table 4.1 *Summary of skills involved in assessment (adapted from Lindberg et al., 1990)*

Assessment	Definition	Tools needed	Example
Observation	Seeing or sensing	Senses	Pallor; bruising; withdrawn state
Interview	Face-to-face or telephone discussion to discuss a particular issue	Communication skills Appropriate environment	Planned conference Informal discussion when providing care
Listening	Purposefully attending to someone	Senses Appropriate environment Communication skills	Recognition of underlying concerns
Consultation	Using additional resources (e.g. tertiary data sources)	Evidence-based practice Inter–professional working	Specialist practitioner to provide additional data
Inspection	Close and purposeful observation	Senses – sight, hearing, touch Tools such as stethoscope	More focused than observation, e.g. focused on specific data, such as blood pressure recording

(continued)

Table 4.1 (*continued*)

Assessment	Definition	Tools needed	Example
Palpation	Use of hands or fingers to examine external surface of the body	Touch Vision	Location of pain Feeling for a pulse
Percussion	Light and sharp tapping on part of the body	Senses – touch, hearing	Location of fluid in a cavity, e.g. fluid on the lungs
Auscultation	Listening with a stethoscope	Hearing	Sounds, such as foetal heartbeat

4.8 Patient involvement in the assessment process

Assessment is key to the processes of care and intervention, and service users' and carers' own assessment of needs and priorities has become increasingly important in health and social care. The focus is on needs-led assessment, with the service user at the centre of the process.

There are often difficulties in pursuing a model of needs-led assessment. These are related to problems of identifying need due to its conceptual complexity (see *Chapter 1*), a historical focus on assessing people for services and the lack of a common framework for assessing needs across professional boundaries.

Neuman (1995) uses a developmental approach to describe the nursing situation and to provide guidance for nursing assessment, and she proposes the use of six broad questions to gain information from the service user:

1. What do you consider to be your major problem, difficulty or area of concern?
2. How has this affected your usual pattern of living or lifestyle?
3. Have you ever experienced a similar problem before? If so, what was that problem and how did you handle it? Was your handling of the problem successful?
4. What do you anticipate for yourself in the future as a consequence of your present situation?
5. What are you doing and what can you do to help yourself?
6. What do you expect care-givers, family, friends and others to do for you?

Although this model was developed for nursing practice, these questions are very general and could be used by any health and social care practitioner to assess an individual's needs and strengths. These questions are also useful as they acknowledge the role of the service user and carers in the caring process and assess service users' own perceptions of their needs and strengths and coping mechanisms. This fits in with the person-centred and individualised approach to care provision, as well as reflecting contemporary theoretical approaches to care delivery as holistic and personalised care and the underpinning theory of the Single Assessment Process.

It is also useful to try to understand what the service user expectation of care is. In initial assessment situations, it could be helpful to think about the acronym ICE:

- Ideas
- Concerns
- Expectations.

Following this outline helps you to understand what ideas the service user has about what the problem might be and what their concerns are. In asking about expectations, it allows an opportunity to set realistic plans.

LIZZIE

If it transpires that Lizzie had a transient ischaemic attack (mini-stroke), she may fear that she had a full stroke and the temporary weakness will be permanent, resulting in her and Frank needing full-time residential care. In asking the questions about ideas, concerns and expectations, it facilitates an open and comprehensive discussion about the future.

The shift in emphasis from health and social care practitioners as experts in the assessment and management of needs to a more person-centred approach, with service users and carers at the centre of the process of assessment, has led to an increase in the use of self-assessment tools in health and social care (Milner and O'Byrne, 2009). These tools can be used by the service user and/or carer in isolation, or can be used as part of a holistic assessment in conjunction with health and social care practitioners. The General Health Questionnaire (available at www.gl-assessment.co.uk/products/general-health-questionnaire-ghq/) is a good example of a self-assessment tool. It asks the individual to rate their own health status using a rating scale to determine how they are feeling in a number of psychological and physical domains that incorporate comparisons with their normal experience. The PHQ-9 assessment tool is a self-administered questionnaire (available at www.mdcalc.com/phq-9-patient-health-questionnaire-9), used within the community to assess an individual's psychological problems. Self-assessment is therefore important for establishing current needs and problems within the wider context of the individual's life and experiences and for identifying needs as they themselves see them. This can also help to identify strengths and coping mechanisms so that interventions can be tailored to those individual needs.

4.9 Tools for assessment

There are numerous assessment tools that aid the objective assessment of problems and needs. In recent years, there has been a move to develop more systematic tools and assessment forms, in line with government priorities in health and social care, to increase the efficiency and effectiveness of provision, based on a sound evidence base. Each organisation will have a preference for certain tools and it is important that you become familiar with what is used in your own organisation.

4.9.1 Initial assessment tools

Some of the better-known assessment tools and forms are listed in *Table 4.2.*

Table 4.2 *Assessment tools in common use*

Tool	When is it used?	What does it help to assess?
Glasgow Coma Scale	Suspected neurological damage	Vital signs
		Level of consciousness
		Physical strength
Waterlow Scale	Risk of pressure ulcers	Risk factors associated with development of pressure ulcers
NEWS2	Early warning system to identify acutely ill patients	Respiratory rate
		Oxygen saturations
		Temperature
		Systolic blood pressure
		Pulse rate
		Level of consciousness
MUST	To identify adults who are malnourished or at risk of malnutrition	Height and weight
		BMI
		Acute disease effect and score
		Measurements of unplanned weight loss
FRAT (Falls Risk Assessment Tool)	When patient has had previous fall or is at risk of falling	Medication effects
		Footwear suitability
		Fluctuating blood pressure
(TILER) Moving and Handling Assessment	For all patients who require some help in mobilising	What is the nature of mobilisation (movement in bed or standing/walking)?
		What can the patient do with some help/encouragement?
		Load – how heavy is the patient and are there other considerations such as amputation or reluctance to comply?
		Environment – is the area safe to handle a patient? Will I be constrained by furniture or medical devices?
		What aids are used (hoist/stand aid etc.)?
Pain assessment tool – relevant for the client group, e.g. children, people with learning disability and/or mental health difficulties. Examples include Universal Assessment Tool, FLACC, Abbey	To establish the degree of pain experienced by the patient who may be unable to describe the pain	How pain is communicated (verbally and non-verbally)
		Interventions to reduce pain and effectiveness of interventions (such as medication, position-changing, relaxation techniques)

We have highlighted a number of these tools below that can be applied to Frank and Lizzie in relation to nutrition/hydration, communication and infection prevention.

Glasgow Coma Scale

The Glasgow Coma Scale (GCS) is used where there is suspected neurological damage and includes assessment of vital signs as well as level of consciousness and physical strength (see www.patient.info/doctor/glasgow-coma-scale-gcs).

LIZZIE

Refer back to the scenario in which Lizzie suddenly collapsed when out shopping. The GCS could be used to establish:

1. **Verbal response**. Is Lizzie able to talk and provide coherent answers? This will establish level of consciousness, i.e. is Lizzie fully conscious and orientated to time and place? Any disorientation or reduced consciousness may indicate that Lizzie banged her head when she fell or that there is an underlying reason for the fall (e.g. high blood pressure, cerebral vascular incident such as a stroke)

Questions that might be asked to assess this are:
What day and date is it?
Who is currently the Prime Minister?
What were you doing when you fell?

2. **Vital signs**. These will provide baseline data to measure any changes, but may also provide important information that indicates an underlying reason for the fall, e.g. low blood pressure.
3. **Motor response**. Lizzie could be asked to raise her arms in the air or move her legs to check whether she can respond to simple commands and whether there is any paralysis of the limbs, which would indicate more serious pathology as a result of an underlying cause or head injury sustained in the fall. If Lizzie had reduced levels of consciousness then physical stimulation would be used to see if there is a normal response involving limb flexion.
4. **Eye opening**. This will assess whether Lizzie is able to spontaneously open her eyes or open them in relation to a physical stimulus, to establish level of consciousness.

Waterlow Scale

The Waterlow Scale (www.judy-waterlow.co.uk/) is a scale devised to assess a service user's risk of getting pressure sores and is used extensively throughout health and social care practice. Within this scale, the practitioner is guided to assess and score a number of social variables and health factors, and then to add up the scores to determine the level of risk (see *Figure 4.3*).

ACTIVITY 4.7 – FRANK

1. From all the information that you have about Frank, use the Waterlow Scale to identify whether he has any level of risk from pressure sores.
2. Compare your assessment with that of other students. How much level of agreement is there between your different assessments?
3. How useful is something like the Waterlow Scale for the objective assessment of needs?

While the Waterlow Scale is not a precise scientific measuring tool, as some of the categories are open to different subjective interpretations, as well as making assumptions based on age and gender groupings, it does guide practitioners in terms of what they should assess and provides an indication of risk to inform care planning and intervention. Tools are useful, but should be used in conjunction with the nurse's own observations and judgements.

NEWS2

The Royal College of Physicians updated the National Early Warning Score (NEWS) in December 2017 to create the NEWS2 scoring system (www.rcplondon.ac.uk/projects/outputs/national-early-warning-score-news-2). This is widely implemented across the UK and it is a track and trigger system to standardise the assessment of acute illness of patients. As you will note, the patient's vital signs are recorded – respiration, oxygen percentage, systolic blood pressure, heart rate, conscious level (which includes new delirium) and temperature (*Figure 4.4*). The normal parameters are clear and when a patient has a recording outside of a normal parameter, there will be a trigger to suggest that further investigation is needed (*Figure 4.5*).

LIZZIE

When Lizzie collapsed in the supermarket, it is likely that the paramedic would assess her using the NEWS2 tool. She would be able to identify quickly whether Lizzie was in a critical condition such as cardiac arrest or whether she may be acutely ill with an infection that could lead to sepsis.

MUST

Another nationally used assessment tool is the Malnutrition Universal Screening Tool (MUST). This is used in most hospital and community settings and helps to assess the patient's nutritional status. The links between poor nutrition and ill health are well established and often patients do not eat well in hospitals. For information about this tool see www.bapen.org.uk/pdfs/must/must_full.pdf. You will see the links between MUST and BMI assessment.

WATERLOW PRESSURE ULCER PREVENTION/TREATMENT POLICY
RING SCORES IN TABLE, ADD TOTAL. MORE THAN 1 SCORE/CATEGORY CAN BE USED

BUILD/WEIGHT FOR HEIGHT	◆	SKIN TYPE VISUAL RISK AREAS	◆	SEX AGE	◆
AVERAGE BMI = 20-24.9	0	HEALTHY	0	MALE	1
ABOVE AVERAGE BMI = 25-29.9	1	TISSUE PAPER	1	FEMALE	2
OBESE BMI > 30	2	DRY	1	14-49	1
BELOW AVERAGE BMI < 20	3	OEDEMATOUS	1	50-64	2
BMI = Wt(Kg)/Ht (m)²		CLAMMY, PYREXIA	1	65-74	3
		DISCOLOURED GRADE 1	2	75-80	4
		BROKEN/SPOTS GRADE 2-4	3	81 +	5

MALNUTRITION SCREENING TOOL (MST) (Nutrition Vol.15, No.6 1999 - Australia) ◆

A - HAS PATIENT LOST WEIGHT RECENTLY		B - WEIGHT LOSS SCORE	
YES	- GO TO B	0.5 - 5 kg	= 1
NO	- GO TO C	5 - 10 kg	= 2
UNSURE	- GO TO C AND SCORE 2	10 - 15 kg	= 3
		>15 kg	= 4
		unsure	= 2

C - PATIENT EATING POORLY OR LACK OF APPETITE	NUTRITION SCORE
'NO' = 0; 'YES' SCORE = 1	If > 2 refer for nutrition assessment/intervention

CONTINENCE	◆	MOBILITY	◆
COMPLETE/ CATHETERISED	0	FULLY	0
URINE INCONT.	1	RESTLESS/FIDGETY	1
FAECAL INCONT.	2	APATHETIC	2
URINARY + FAECAL INCONTINENCE	3	RESTRICTED	3
		BEDBOUND e.g. TRACTION	4
		CHAIRBOUND e.g. WHEELCHAIR	5

SPECIAL RISKS

TISSUE MALNUTRITION	◆	NEUROLOGICAL DEFICIT	◆
TERMINAL CACHEXIA	8	DIABETES, MS, CVA	4-6
MULTIPLE ORGAN FAILURE	8	MOTOR/SENSORY	4-6
SINGLE ORGAN FAILURE (RESP, RENAL, CARDIAC.)	5	PARAPLEGIA (MAX OF 6)	4-6
PERIPHERAL VASCULAR DISEASE	5		
ANAEMIA (Hb <8)	2		
SMOKING	1		

MAJOR SURGERY or TRAUMA	
ORTHOPAEDIC/SPINAL	5
ON TABLE > 2 HR#	5
ON TABLE > 6 HR#	8

MEDICATION - CYTOTOXICS, LONG TERM/HIGH DOSE STEROIDS, ANTI-INFLAMMATORY   MAX OF 4

Scores can be discounted after 48 hours provided patient is recovering normally

SCORE

10+ AT RISK
15+ HIGH RISK
20+ VERY HIGH RISK

© J Waterlow 1985 Revised 2005*

www.judy-waterlow.co.uk

Obtainable from the Nook, Stoke Road, Henlade TAUNTON TA3 5LX

The 2005 revision incorporates the research undertaken by Queensland Health.

Figure 4.3 The Waterlow Scale.

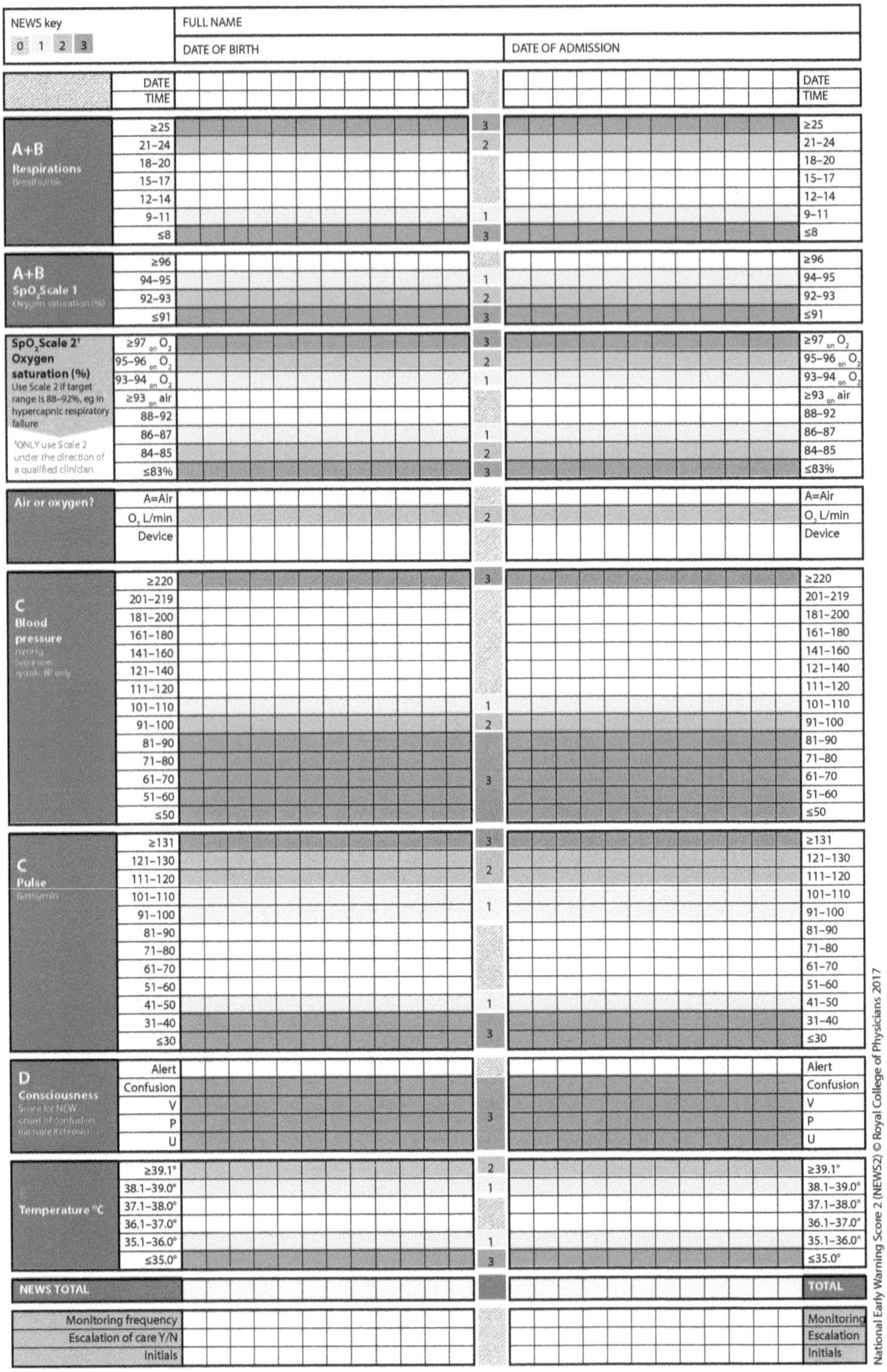

NEWS key	FULL NAME		
0 1 2 3	DATE OF BIRTH		DATE OF ADMISSION

		DATE												DATE
		TIME												TIME

A+B Respirations (Breaths/min)

	Score
≥25	3
21–24	2
18–20	
15–17	
12–14	
9–11	1
≤8	3

A+B SpO₂ Scale 1 (Oxygen saturation (%))

	Score
≥96	
94–95	1
92–93	2
≤91	3

SpO₂ Scale 2† Oxygen saturation (%) Use Scale 2 if target range is 88–92%, eg in hypercapnic respiratory failure. †ONLY use Scale 2 under the direction of a qualified clinician

	Score
≥97 on O₂	3
95–96 on O₂	2
93–94 on O₂	1
≥93 on air	
88–92	
86–87	1
84–85	2
≤83%	3

Air or oxygen?

	Score
A=Air	
O₂ L/min	2
Device	

C Blood pressure mmHg. Score uses systolic BP only

	Score
≥220	3
201–219	
181–200	
161–180	
141–160	
121–140	
111–120	
101–110	1
91–100	2
81–90	
71–80	
61–70	3
51–60	
≤50	

C Pulse (Beats/min)

	Score
≥131	3
121–130	2
111–120	
101–110	
91–100	1
81–90	
71–80	
61–70	
51–60	
41–50	1
31–40	
≤30	3

D Consciousness Score for NEW onset of confusion (no score if chronic)

	Score
Alert	
Confusion	
V	3
P	
U	

Temperature °C

	Score
≥39.1°	2
38.1–39.0°	1
37.1–38.0°	
36.1–37.0°	
35.1–36.0°	1
≤35.0°	3

NEWS TOTAL	

Monitoring frequency	
Escalation of care Y/N	
Initials	

National Early Warning Score 2 (NEWS2) © Royal College of Physicians 2017

Figure 4.4 NEWS2 observation chart.
Reproduced from: Royal College of Physicians (2017). *National Early Warning Score (NEWS) 2: Standardising the assessment of acute-illness severity in the NHS*. Updated report of a working party. London, 2017. Available from: www.rcplondon.ac.uk/projects/outputs/national-early-warning-score-news-2.

Aggregate score 0–4	Low	Ward-based response
Red score Score of 3 in any individual parameter	Low–medium	Urgent ward-based response*
Aggregate score 5–6	Medium	Key threshold for urgent response*
Aggregate score 7 or more	High	Urgent or emergency response**

Figure 4.5 *NEWS2 thresholds and triggers.*
Reproduced from: Royal College of Physicians (2017). *National Early Warning Score (NEWS) 2: Standardising the assessment of acute-illness severity in the NHS*. Updated report of a working party. London, 2017. Available from: www.rcplondon.ac.uk/projects/outputs/national-early-warning-score-news-2.
*Response by a clinician or team with competence in the assessment and treatment of acutely ill patients and in recognising when the escalation of care to a critical care team is appropriate.
**The response team must also include staff with critical care skills, including airway management.

FRANK

If you apply this tool to Frank, it is likely that his score would show that he is not eating sufficient calories and protein. His score would show that his health is deteriorating and that a plan to increase his nutritional intake is needed. The advice from the dietetic department, in conjunction with medical staff, would therefore be incorporated into his care plan.

As well as the nutritional status assessment, it is usual for a patient's hydration to be observed. There are numerous tools to do this and each organisation will have its own version (see *Figure 4.6*). Essentially, these tools measure the amount of fluid a person takes in and the volume of fluid excreted. It is worth remembering that not all fluid is taken by drinking. You would have to include intake such as soup or intravenous/subcutaneous therapy. In a critical care area, total parenteral nutrition (TPN) would also be measured. The most common rationale for measuring how much fluid a patient takes in is when a patient has a cardiac problem or renal difficulties. The fluid lost each day would also be measured and again, it is not just urine output that would be considered; if a patient had diarrhoea or is sweating profusely, this would be taken into account. In a critical care environment, a faecal catheter might be used to measure output.

LIZZIE

When Lizzie is admitted to hospital following her collapse, a fluid balance chart would be used to assess the balance. A quick initial assessment of hydration would be to look at the state of her tongue and the back of her hands, which is a quick and easy thing to do. Often the tongue and skin on the back of a patient's hand can show hydration levels, as the tongue will be dry and the skin will stay pinched instead of becoming smooth quickly. If Lizzie is not drinking sufficiently, it is likely that her tongue will be dry and it may become 'furred' or develop cracks in it.

NHS

| Name: |
| Address: |
| DOB: |
| CRN/Hospital No: |
| NHS Number: |

Fluid Balance Chart

Ward: _____   Consultant: _____   Patient's weight: _____

Date Commenced: _____   Refer to Guidelines if chart is predominantly used for input only (e.g. Rehab)

Time	Intake: ml			Other		Running total	Output: ml		Other (chest drain, etc)			Running total	Initials
	Oral	IV (1)	IV (2)				Urine*	NG	Vomit	Bowels			
24.00													
01.00													
02.00													
03.00													
04.00													
05.00	**Patient admitted to the ward here**												
06.00		1000								+			
07.00	SIPS						Pu'D	++		++			
08.00									++				
09.00	SIPS									+			
10.00	**Patient is being seen around now...**												
11.00													
12.00													
13.00													
14.00													
15.00													
16.00													
17.00													
18.00													
19.00													
20.00													
21.00													
22.00													
23.00													
Final Totals													

Total Intake **(A)**	Output Measurement			Balance (A–D)
	Output (B)	Insensible Loss **(C)** 600 ml or Calculated:_____	**Total Output (D)** (B&C Added)	This must not be left blank

Low urine output triggers EWS 4+ if patients are having hourly urine measurement and urine output is less than 30 ml/hr for 3 hours in a row OR if the patient is catheterised and urine output is found to be less than 129 ml on four hourly emptying

Figure 4.6 *Example of a fluid balance chart.*

NHS

North Tees and Hartlepool
NHS Foundation Trust

| Name: |
| Address: |
| DOB: |
| CRN/Hospital No: |
| NHS Number: |

Food and Fluid Monitoring Care Plan

Day 1 - Date: ....

Please record the type and amount of food and drinks offered and consumed.

	Description of food and drink provided	Portion size			Amount taken						Fluid consumed (mls)	Initial
		S	M	L	Declined	None	¼	½	¾	All		
Breakfast												
	Action and comments											
Mid morning												
	Action and comments											
Lunch												
	Action and comments											
Mid afternoon												
	Action and comments											
Evening meal												
	Action and comments											
Supper												
	Action and comments											
Night time												
	Action and comments											
Total fluid (mls) consumed in 24 hours:												
	Action and comments											

Figure 4.7 *Example of food and fluid monitoring form.*

NHS

North Tees and Hartlepool
NHS Foundation Trust

Food and Fluid Monitoring Care Plan
To be completed for all meals, snacks and drinks

Name:
Address:
DOB:
CRN/Hospital No:
NHS Number:

Right Nutrition Every Time

Complete checklist daily	Day Initial when completed							
	Day	1	2	*3	4	5	6	*7
	Date and time							
• Offer 2 nourishing snacks daily *Where swallowing problems exist check snacks are correct consistency.*								
• Offer milky drinks or nourishing drinks *Where swallowing problems exist check drinks are correct consistency.*								
• Moderate risk*: provide 3 cups of full cream milk daily *Where swallowing problems exist check drinks are correct consistency.*								
• High risk*: Ensure patient is referred to Dietitian **Initial when complete.** *While swallowing problems exist consider referral to SALT.*								
• Use a red tray at mealtimes *If patient requires assistance.*								
• Complete food and fluid record charts for meals, snacks and drinks								
• Complete *3 or *7 day review of food and fluid record charts								

Figure 4.7 *Example of food and fluid monitoring form (continued).*
Reproduced with permission from North Tees and Hartlepool NHS Foundation Trust.
*Moderate and high risk categories document N/A, if not applicable.

It may also be useful to monitor food intake, especially if the patient has been assessed as malnourished or at risk of malnutrition. Again, each Trust will have its own version, but *Figure 4.7* shows how food intake could be recorded.

Pain assessment tools

Some tools can be standardised or become universally adopted but there is often a need to have a bespoke type of assessment tool. An example would be when trying to assess a person's pain. Communication is necessary when assessing pain and not all patients communicate verbally so adaptations are needed.

4.9.2 FLACC pain scale

For example, think back to Stacey in *Chapter 3*, who has a learning difficulty and may not always clearly communicate pain. Using a tool such as a FLACC pain scale may be appropriate. This scale is used to observe Face, Legs, Activity, Cry, Consolability (FLACC) (see www.health.gov.au/internet/publications/publishing.nsf/Content/triageqrg~triageqrg-pain~triageqrg-FLACC).

This scale (*Table 4.3*) has five criteria, each of which is scored 0, 1 or 2, giving a total score of 0 to 10.

Table 4.3 *FLACC pain scale*

Criteria	Score 0	Score 1	Score 2
Face	No particular expression or smile	Occasional grimace or frown, withdrawn, uninterested	Frequent to constant quivering chin, clenched jaw
Legs	Normal position or relaxed	Uneasy, restless, tense	Kicking, or legs drawn up
Activity	Lying quietly, normal position, moves easily	Squirming, shifting, back and forth, tense	Arched, rigid or jerking
Cry	No cry (awake or asleep)	Moans or whimpers; occasional complaint	Crying steadily, screams or sobs, frequent complaints
Consolability	Content, relaxed	Reassured by occasional touching, hugging or being talked to, distractible	Difficult to console or comfort

4.9.3 The Abbey Pain Scale

In the case of Frank, he has some cognitive impairment and may not easily verbalise pain. There are numerical assessment tools (to give the pain a number between 1 and 10) and visual assessment tools (where faces vary between smiles and frowns) but the Abbey Pain Scale (*Figure 4.8*) is specifically designed for people with dementia. This tool helps to assess:

- VOCALISATION, e.g. crying, groaning and whimpering
- FACIAL EXPRESSION, e.g. looking tense, frowning, grimacing, looking frightened
- CHANGES IN BODY LANGUAGE, e.g. fidgeting, rocking, guarding part of the body and withdrawal
- BEHAVIOURAL CHANGE, e.g. increased confusion, refusing to eat, alteration in usual patterns
- PHYSIOLOGICAL CHANGES, e.g. temperature, pulse or blood pressure, flushing, pallor
- PHYSICAL CHANGES, e.g. skin tears, pressure areas, arthritis contractures, previous injuries.

Each category is given a rating of Absent, Mild, Moderate or Severe on a 0–3 scale and a total score given.

Abbey Pain Scale

For measurement of pain in people with dementia who cannot verbalise.

How to use scale: While observing the resident, score questions 1 to 6

Name of resident: ....

Name and designation of person completing the scale: ....

Date: .... **Time:** ....

Latest pain relief given was .... at .... hrs.

Q1. Vocalisation
   e.g. whimpering, groaning, crying   **Q1** [   ]
   Absent 0   Mild 1   Moderate 2   Severe 3

Q2. Facial expression
   e.g. looking tense, frowning, grimacing, looking frightened   **Q2** [   ]
   Absent 0   Mild 1   Moderate 2   Severe 3

Q3. Change in body language
   e.g. fidgeting, rocking, guarding part of body, withdrawn   **Q3** [   ]
   Absent 0   Mild 1   Moderate 2   Severe 3

Q4. Behavioural change
   e.g. increased confusion, refusing to eat, alteration in usual patterns   **Q4** [   ]
   Absent 0   Mild 1   Moderate 2   Severe 3

Q5. Physiological change
   e.g. temperature, pulse or blood pressure outside normal limits,   **Q5** [   ]
   perspiring, flushing or pallor
   Absent 0   Mild 1   Moderate 2   Severe 3

Q6. Physical changes
   e.g. skin tears, pressure areas, arthritis, contractures,   **Q6** [   ]
   previous injuries
   Absent 0   Mild 1   Moderate 2   Severe 3

Add scores for 1–6 and record here   ⟹   **Total Pain Score** [   ]

Now tick the box that matches
the Total Pain score   ⟹

0–2	3–7	8–13	14+
No pain	**Mild**	**Moderate**	**Severe**

Finally, tick the box which matches
the type of pain   ⟹

Chronic	Acute	Acute on Chronic

Dementia Care Australia Pty Ltd
Website: www.dementiacareaustralia.com

Figure 4.8 *The Abbey Pain Scale.*
Abbey, J., De Bellis, A., Piller, N., Esterman, A., Giles, L., Parker, D. and Lowcay, B. Funded by the J.H. & J.D. Gunn Medical Research Foundation 1998–2002.

Other assessment tools

Depending on the context and reason that someone needs healthcare attention, there are other specific tools to consider such as:
- depression/delirium/dementia (HAD or GAD)
- frailty assessment
- falls risk assessment.

ACTIVITY 4.8

Talk to your practice supervisor and identify which tools are used locally related to depression, frailty and falls risk.

4.9.4 Secondary assessment tools

Secondary assessment tools might be considered for use within 24–48 hours of admission.

Spiritual assessment

An example is the spiritual assessment SPIR, developed by Frick *et al.* (2006). This tool requires the assessment of four characteristics:
- S: Would you describe yourself as a believing, **s**piritual or religious person?
- P: What is the **p**lace of spirituality in your life and in the context of your illness?
- I: Are you **i**ntegrated in a spiritual community?
- R: What **r**ole would you like to assign to your nurse in the domain of spirituality?

Assessment of cultural dimension

Another secondary assessment tool might be to determine the cultural dimension of the patient. The need to provide culturally competent care is an important requirement in light of the *Future Nurse* standards (NMC, 2018b) identified in Platform 2: Promoting and preventing ill health. There are various assessment tools but the Sunrise Enabler by Madeleine Leininger (Leininger and McFarland, 2005) is of particular interest (www.madeleine-leininger.com/resources.shtml). This tool (*Figure 4.9*) tries to establish the patient's world view and assesses seven factors:
- Technological
- Religious/philosophical
- Kinship/social
- Cultural values/beliefs/lifeways
- Political and legal
- Economical
- Educational.

ACTIVITY 4.9 – Frank

Can you use the 'Sunrise Enabler' tool shown in *Figure 4.9* to assess Frank's cultural perspective? Look at the factors and use information you have about Frank to try to identify his spiritual beliefs and his attitude to healthcare. What influences Frank's world view?

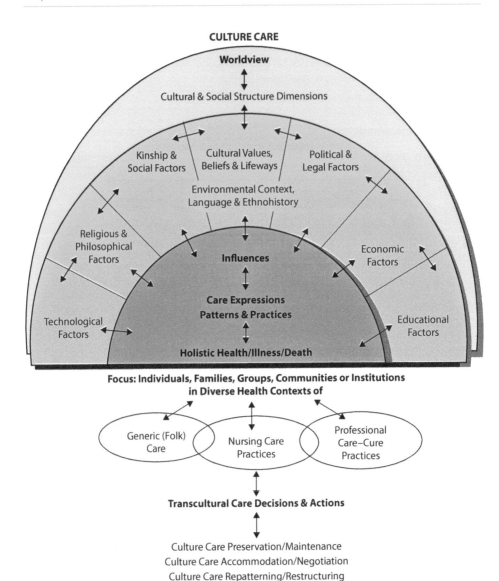

Figure 4.9 *Sunrise Enabler Diagram.*
Reproduced under a Creative Commons Attribution 4.0 International Licence.

4.9.5 Holistic assessment tools

A more holistic assessment tool might guide the practitioner and service user
to assess the current situation in the context of wider social, environmental and
ecological variables. For example, genograms and life road maps are used as tools to
help identify needs. Genograms are a modified family tree and provide a snapshot
of the individual's family and how the service user views it at that particular time

(see *Figure 4.10*). These are fairly simple to produce but may provide a powerful tool for the exploration of family relationships or identification of life crises that have impacted on the individual.

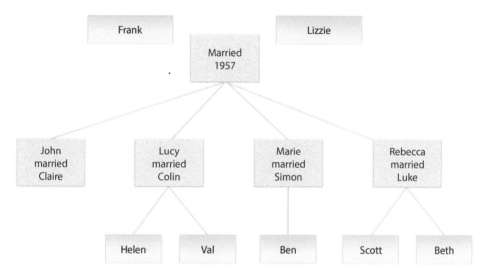

Figure 4.10 *Frank and Lizzie's family genogram (simple).*

A practitioner could use this as a guide to establish the informal care network that Frank and Lizzie have and establish whether any relatives are able to provide physical and/or emotional support as part of a holistic package of care provision. For example, using this simple genogram, we might establish whether any of the children and/or grandchildren live nearby and are able to drive Frank and Lizzie to the shops or clinical appointments. Genograms are particularly useful when assessing children, to look at the different interrelationships that a child may have and where the risk and protective relationships are.

Dahlgren–Whitehead model

A more comprehensive holistic assessment tool was developed by Dahlgren and Whitehead in 1991. They identify layers of influence on individual health, as in a rainbow. They describe a social ecological theory to health and attempt to show the relationship between the individual, their environment and disease (*Figure 4.11*). The individual is at the centre with a set of fixed genes, surrounded by influences on health that can be modified. For example, personal behaviour and lifestyle choices can promote or damage health. If, for instance, smoking is seen as antisocial by a community or group of people, the perceived disapproval may affect the smoker's relationships with others. The next layer, social and community influences, may provide support for members of the community in unfavourable conditions, but may also provide no support or have a negative effect. The third layer includes structural factors, such as housing, working conditions, access to services and provision of essential facilities.

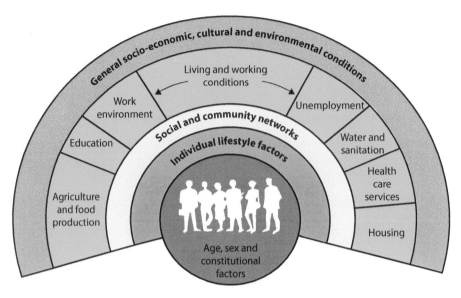

Figure 4.11 *The Dahlgren–Whitehead rainbow. Reproduced with permission from Institute for Futures Studies.*

ACTIVITY 4.10 - FRANK AND LIZZIE

Go back to the case study of Frank and Lizzie and use the categories from Dahlgren and Whitehead's model in *Figure 4.11* to identify the influences on their health.

4.9.6 Assessing children

There are very clear differences between assessing adults and assessing children so as a starting point, it would be good to consider some of the main difficulties. For example, communication – what barriers are there to communicating with children? Think about the age continuum. If a child has pain, how would you know? If a child needs an intervention such as an injection, how do you gain consent? Children may also have other issues such as a learning difficulty or mental health problem to take into account. There is the additional complication of considering the care-giver's perspectives and needs – this could be the parent or any adult who is with the child. The assessment is multifaceted and it is not a straightforward 'one person to another' communication event.

The Healthy Child Programme (2018) provides evidence to support children in the UK. Public Health England (2018) has also set guidance documents for health visitors and children's nurses to promote good health for people aged 0 to 19 and to recognise and intervene when good health is not apparent (see also www.gov.uk/government/publications/healthy-child-programme-pregnancy-and-the-first-5-years-of-life).

This should be read in conjunction with the World Health Organization (WHO) Child Growth Standards (WHO/United Nations Children's Fund, 2009), which identify severe acute malnutrition in infants and children (www.who.int/childgrowth/en/).

Jonathan is an eight-week-old healthy baby who has been achieving milestones and thriving. Helen has been feeding him with formula milk as she did not like the thought of breastfeeding. She is with James and they hope to get married next year. Helen is on maternity leave from her job as a shop assistant.

Helen is a bit concerned about her baby as he has been 'snuffly' for the last few days and is not taking his feeds as well as he was. Jonathan also feels hot to the touch and the digital thermometer she used recorded a temperature of 37.2°C. She has given him the recommended dose of paediatric paracetamol which has helped to settle him so he takes his feeds and sleeps well, which he did last night. Helen does not know whether to take him for his immunisation appointment due tomorrow.

How might you advise Helen?

This chapter has focused on the assessment stage of the process of care (ASPIRE). Building on *Chapters 1* to *3*, which set the historical and policy context, it has explored the contemporary nature of assessment at the beginning of the 21st century. The nature of assessment and the essential nature of communication and other skills within the ASPIRE process were discussed. By examining the purpose of assessment, different approaches and tools of assessment and the contemporary focus on self-assessment, the student of health and social care will be able to articulate the reasons and rationale for undertaking assessments in health and social care. Subjective and objective approaches to assessment have been discussed and the benefits of each examined. Tools for assessment have also been identified and their benefits discussed within the changing nature of health and social care and the contested notion of the expert in assessment of need when considering the context of the service user's and carer's lives.

Reflection

Identify at least three things that you have learned from this chapter.	1. .... 2. .... 3. ....
How do you plan to use this knowledge within clinical practice?	1. .... 2. .... 3. ....

How will you evaluate the
effectiveness of your plan?

1. ....

....

2. ....

....

3. ....

....

What further knowledge and
evidence do you need?

1. ....

....

2. ....

....

3. ....

....

Further Reading

Standing, M. (2017) *Clinical Judgement and Decision Making for Nursing Students*, 3rd edition. Exeter: Learning Matters.

This book provides a comprehensive discussion of theoretical issues in relation to clinical decision-making. The book is based on research findings about student nurses' perceptions of decision-making, exploring a wide range of clinical nursing decisions throughout the patient journey. There are chapters on collaborative and standardised decision-making, systematic decision-making, ethical decision-making, observation, prioritising care delivery, experience and intuition, reflective judgement, accountability and confidence. Throughout the book, case studies and activities help the reader to apply the theories to practice.

Foot, C., Gilburt, H., Dunn, P. *et al.* (2014) *People in Control of their own Health and Care: the state of involvement.* The King's Fund in association with National Voices. Available from: www.kingsfund.org.uk/sites/default/files/field/field_publication_file/people-in-control-of-their-own-health-and-care-the-state-of-involvement-november-2014.pdf) (accessed 22 April 2019)

This paper should make nurses think about how we 'put patients first'. The art of assessment is about trying to understand from a patient what the issue is and how we can help to make the best assessment of what to do to help. This document helps to see the importance of authentic involvement of service users in their care and treatment.

Paediatric Early Warning Score: PEWS at www.clinicalguidelines.scot.nhs.uk/ggc-paediatric-guidelines/ggc-guidelines/surgery/paediatric-early-warning-score-pews/

This is an essential read for anyone who is involved in the assessment of children who are acutely ill. The document covers assessment of end-of-life care, sepsis, neurological and pain assessment.

Chapter 5
Planning

LEARNING OUTCOMES

This chapter will cover the following key issues:

- The nature of planning care and support

- Goal setting and SMART objectives

- Partnership working within the multidisciplinary team

- Collaborative working with service users and carers

- The importance of keeping accurate written records and confidentiality

- The financial aspects of care planning.

By the end of this chapter you should be able to:

- discuss the importance of the planning phase of the care process

- apply the principles of care planning to practice

- articulate the practitioner's role in working in partnership with other health and social care practitioners

- discuss the nature of working in collaboration for integrated care.

While many elements of the NMC platforms that make up the standards of proficiency for registered nurses are covered, this chapter has particular reference to (NMC, 2018b):

- Platform 3: Assessing needs and planning care

- Platform 7: Coordinating care

For further detailed mapping please see *Appendix 1* – Detailed mapping to *Future Nurse: standards of proficiency for registered nurses*.

5.1 Introduction

Planning is the second phase of the ASPIRE cycle (*Figure 5.1*).

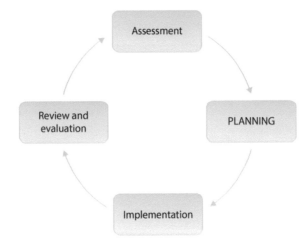

Figure 5.1 *The planning phase of the ASPIRE cycle.*

Although assessment is the cornerstone of good-quality care, planning of appropriate interventions is also fundamental to the care process and patient experience. The planning phase of the care process involves the development of strategies to reduce, minimise or address the problem or need that was identified in the assessment phase of the process. This consists of four stages (Howatson-Jones *et al.*, 2015):

1. Setting priorities
2. Developing outcomes
3. Developing orders (measures or interventions)
4. Documentation.

These stages of planning are important in all healthcare encounters, but in managing the care of someone with complex needs and/or a long-term condition, it is particularly important to identify the priorities of need and support and to develop realistic outcomes, which can be effectively evaluated. Just as assessment is an ongoing process, so the planning phase involves a staged and ongoing systematic process.

Care pathways and protocols are frequently used in healthcare to give a consistent and evidence-based plan of care to service users. A care pathway is a standardised plan of care that a 'typical' patient would follow. For example, if an older adult who is normally fit and healthy fell and sustained a fracture to her hip, she could adhere to a prescribed plan of care with the expectation that she would have routine pre-operative care, surgery and post-operative care followed by rehabilitation and discharge. There are examples of care pathways later in this chapter.

Some aspects of care are applicable to all patients, such as 'intentional rounding'. This is where all patients will be seen by a member of the care team at least once an hour. This was introduced so that patients would not have to request assistance by using a call bell; instead they could expect a healthcare practitioner to see them at least once in every hour.

5.1.1 REEPIG

REEPIG is a tool you can apply to ensure that a plan or intervention is realistic, explicit, evidence-based, prioritised, involved and goal-centred (adapted from Hogston, 2011, pp. 2–21):

- To ensure your plan is **Realistic** it is important to consider whether the care can be given within the available resources or practical constraints such as physical availability, otherwise it will not be achievable.
- An **Explicit** plan ensures that statements are qualified so there is no room for misinterpretation. For example, when planning a dressing change state exactly when or the exact circumstances that indicate change is required.
- Plans must be **Evidence-based** as nursing is a research-based profession to ensure care is effective. Research findings that underpin the rationale for care must be considered.
- **Prioritised** plans mean that we start with the most pressing diagnosis. The first priority may be, for example, to plan care for the client's pain.
- The plan of care should **Involve** not only the client, but also the other members of the healthcare team who when working collaboratively can improve outcomes, for example physiotherapists and dietitians.
- Plans must finally be **Goal-centred** to ensure that the care planned meets the outcomes needed.

5.2 Goal setting

Goal setting is an important part of the planning process, and involves predictions about what the care recipient hopes to achieve through the planned interventions. Goals should aim to develop an individual's strengths so that they feel in control of the situation and can share in the problem-solving approach to care. Goals are often written in behavioural terms and should be person-centred to address individual needs. They should also state who expects to attain the result. It is also important when setting goals that the goals are measurable and achievable, and have specific criteria stated to measure the outcome of the planned intervention. The establishment of goals that are measurable enables care to be evaluated and then improved upon (Hambridge and McEwing, 2009).

SMART objectives are useful when setting goals and should be:
- **S**pecific
- **M**easurable
- **A**chievable
- **R**ealistic
- **T**ime-bound.

For example, if you were caring for a patient with a pressure ulcer, you could plan for the sacral ulcer (specific) to reduce from a diameter of 5 mm to a diameter of 3 mm (measurable) within two weeks (time-bound) as long as the patient continues to comply with the dressing regime and consumes a nutritional diet, and continues with two-hourly positional changes (achievable and realistic).

It is also worth considering that goals may be 'stretch' goals, meaning that the patient will become more enabled or better at performing a function. Often in rehabilitation situations, the goal might be to maintain a certain level of function or ability. For example, a person with Parkinson's disease or any other progressive illness might set a goal to maintain a current level of independence and mobility.

ACTIVITY 5.1: FRANK

Refer back to Lizzie and Frank's story.

Imagine you are the Mental Health Nurse who has been assigned to Frank's case. What SMART plan can you put in place to address his low mood?

Another way of setting goals is to ensure that they conform to the MACROS criteria (Hogston, 2007). These are goals that are:

- **M**easurable (and observable so that the outcome can be evaluated)
- **A**chievable and time-limited
- **C**lient-centred
- **R**ealistic
- **O**utcome-written
- **S**hort.

Consider the example for the patient with a sacral pressure ulcer. How would you write the plan using MACROS?

ACTIVITY 5.2

Think about a learning need that you have. For example, you may need to learn to drive or to learn how to make medication calculations. Develop a plan, using SMART or MACROS objectives, to determine what you want to achieve, how you are going to achieve it and how you are going to measure the level of achievement.

Some needs are complex and may require the development of a number of SMART or MACROS objectives, with short-, medium- and long-term goals. This is what is meant by being realistic. If a goal is too ambitious (not realistic) it can be demoralising, as the individual is unable to see how they can achieve that goal.

ACTIVITY 5.3

Scott is Frank and Lizzie's grandson. He has been overweight since early childhood and hated PE and games at school as he always felt very self-conscious about his body and quickly got out of breath on exertion, making it difficult to perform in team sports and competitive games. Scott has therefore got used to leading a sedentary lifestyle and has used food as a way of comforting himself as he has become increasingly lonely and socially isolated. He is now 26 years old and weighs 32 stone (just over 200 kg). He has now admitted that he needs to lose weight in order to not only feel that he can participate more actively in society, but also to prevent further health damage and premature mortality.

Using SMART or MACROS objectives, devise a plan of care to help Scott achieve his long-term goal of losing half his body weight.

5.3 Integrated care

Care planning involves the notion of partnership working, collaboration and joined-up thinking. Statutory frameworks and guidance have emphasised partnership and collaborative working since the inception of the modernisation framework for health and social care services in 1998 (Department of Health, 1997 and 1998). Professional codes of practice emphasise the centrality of partnership working to good-quality care.

Health and social care professionals are now educated in 'inter-professional learning' but also in terms of seeing working with clients as a type of partnership.

5.3.1 What is partnership?

For practitioners in health and social care it is impossible not to work with other people in the daily working environment. In the context of contemporary health and social care, working in partnership involves working with other health and social care professionals in the multidisciplinary team, as well as with service users and carers. Collaborative working involves working with service users and carers to identify the problems that need to be addressed and the best way to address them.

Partnership working is therefore seen as beneficial and desirable as it can (Hatton, 2008):

- improve the effectiveness of the care and support process
- see service users and carers as a source of knowledge and understanding, which is fundamental to person-centred and individualised care
- ensure that service user and carer rights remain central to the decision-making process
- facilitate the process of empowerment for service users and carers.

The NHS is committed to reducing inequalities of access and outcome in healthcare and to promoting secure integrated care where it will improve the quality of services (Health and Social Care Act, Department of Health, 2012a).

Collaborative working involves working jointly with each other, reflecting concepts of empowerment and anti-oppressive practice (Carnwell and Buchanan, 2005). Partnerships therefore can be about contractual arrangements, whilst collaboration is about the nature of the partnership and implies a shared agenda, vision and goals.

Ingredients for successful partnership with both other professionals and service users include:
- trust and respect
- shared expertise (it is important to remember that the service user is expert in their lived experience)
- leadership
- participation – non-hierarchical
- shared responsibility and willingness to work together
- strategies to overcome barriers
- communication.

5.3.2 Types of partnership

Partnership and collaborative working are not new to healthcare, but have been widely promoted as a desirable way to work to address needs and solve problems. Whittington (2003) identifies three broad ways that working in an integrated partnership might operate:
1. Agencies working together to provide joined-up services (such as voluntary agencies and housing).
2. Meeting service user needs through the provision of services by more than one organisation (e.g. crossing the boundaries between health and social care agencies, statutory and independent care providers and private organisations).
3. A collaborative relationship between care provider and the service user and carer.

Increasingly, care is provided in multidisciplinary teams who have a shared purpose in delivering person-centred care, as set out by NHS England (2015).

As a nurse you will be working in multidisciplinary teams, which will include some or all of the following:
- Patients and informal carers
- Medical practitioners
- Professions allied to medicine (e.g. physiotherapists, dietitians, occupational therapists, podiatrists)
- Statutory organisations such as schools
- Social care practitioners (e.g. social workers, formal care workers)
- Private healthcare organisations
- Volunteers

- Religious advisors
- Ancillary staff
- Advocate staff
- Interpreters.

The focus on person-centred care and collaborative working reflects a power shift, where service users are seen as active contributors to every stage of the ASPIRE process. This is known as co-production, and its key elements are as follows (Social Care Institute for Excellence, 2013):

- It emphasises that people are not passive recipients of services and have assets and expertise, which can help improve services.
- It is a potentially transformative way of thinking about power, resources, partnerships, risks and outcomes, not an off-the-shelf model of service provision or a single magic solution.
- It focuses on empowerment of both users and providers to act as partners in the care process. Co-production means involving citizens in collaborative relationships with more empowered front line staff who are able and confident to share power and accept user expertise.
- Staff should be trained in the benefits of co-production, supported in positive risk-taking and encouraged to identify new opportunities for collaboration with people who use services.
- People should be encouraged to access co-productive initiatives, recognising and supporting diversity among the people who use services.
- The creation of new structures, regulatory and commissioning practices and financial streams is necessary to embed co-production as a long-term rather than an ad hoc solution.
- Learning from existing international case studies of co-production while recognising the contribution of initiatives reflecting local needs is important.

5.3.3 Integrated care

The NHS faces huge financial pressures due to rising costs and an ageing population with more complex health and social care needs, as discussed in *Chapter 1*. One solution to this is the focus on integrated care, where hospital and community services work together to address the needs of local populations, as set out in the 5-year plan NHS Five Year Forward View in 2014, setting out the road map for integrated care services: "Our aim is to use the next several years to make the biggest national move to integrated care of any major western country" (NHS England, 2017, p. 31).

Partnerships exist between health and social care agencies through joint agreements about the planning and delivery of services, as well as joint commissioning processes. Partnerships also exist in relation to local consultation exercises, where local authorities or the government seek to find out the views of service users and carers in line with the policy agenda to improve service user and carer involvement in decision-making processes at every level of care planning and delivery (see *Chapter 3*). This may be in relation to a specific issue or service, at either a micro or macro level. For example:

- At a micro level, the residents of a care home may be consulted about a change in the social events programme within the home.
- At a macro level people may be consulted about a particular area of need. An example of this might be of a specialist service, such as residential drug and alcohol treatment services within a particular locality.

5.3.4 Barriers to working in partnership

ACTIVITY 5.4

Think about a group or team that you have worked in.

What difficulties did you encounter in working together?

How might group work be sabotaged (either intentionally or unintentionally)?

While there are examples of good partnership working throughout the healthcare sector, there are also a number of barriers to effective partnership working:

- fear of loss of professional identity when working collaboratively with other health and social care practitioners, as well as
- fear of loss of professional identity when working collaboratively with patients and carers (Hudson, 2002)
- lack of integration between different management and organisational structures.

Smale *et al.* (1993) promote the exchange model of working as an effective way of working in partnership with patients and carers. Within this model, it is assumed that people are experts in themselves, while in relation to practitioners it assumes that they (Smale *et al.*, 1993, p. 18):

- have expertise in the process of problem-solving with others
- understand and share perceptions of problems with their management
- will get agreement about who will do what to support whom
- will take responsibility for arriving at the optimum resolution of problems within the constraints of available resources and the willingness of participants to contribute.

ACTIVITY 5.5

Think about how you would feel if you had experience of an issue and were engaging in conversation with someone who did not have your experience but wanted to tell you all about it. Have you ever experienced talking with someone who thinks they have all the answers? It is uncomfortable and you are likely to 'switch off' and disengage from the conversation. Consider the section about communication and how that links to the relationship between patient and care-givers.

Patients who have long-term conditions such as chronic obstructive pulmonary disease are able to attend a course to become an Expert Patient, which addresses the following aims (see www.patient.info/doctor/expert-patients and www.selfmanagementuk.org):

- Setting goals
- Writing an action plan
- Problem-solving skills
- Fitness and exercise
- Better breathing (participants are taught diaphragmatic breathing)
- Fatigue management
- Healthy eating
- Relaxation skills
- Communication with family
- Working better with healthcare professionals, including communicating more effectively with them
- Making better use of medications.

Effective collaborative and partnership working also depends on good record-keeping and addressing issues of confidentiality.

5.4 Writing care plans and keeping records

Care plans relate to the organisation of care that is to be given to an individual client. It is an essential part of the care journey. The care plan is therefore a fundamental tool in health and social care for signposting and agreeing how care is going to be provided. Good practice in relation to record-keeping is important to quality care because the care plan is a written record that is available to everyone involved in the provision of care. Imagine that you are working your first shift with a group of patients – without the care plan, you would have no idea what you should be doing in order to provide continuity of care based on sound assessments.

5.4.1 Key elements of the care plan

There are different ways to record decision-making and care planning. Standardised tools exist to guide practitioners to give the best care. *Table 5.1* shows an example of a care plan that has been standardised for individuals at risk of delirium (see also *Figure 5.2*).

Table 5.1 *Example of a standardised care plan*

Care plan number:	Title: Delirium management and prevention		
Problem:	**Goal(s)**:		
At risk of developing delirium	To reduce risk and promote recovery		
Plan of nursing care:		**Start date**	**End date**
Review cognition daily and report changes to medical staff			
Do you think (patient name) has been more confused or withdrawn today?			
Treat clinical cause			
Consider capacity (refusals of clinical care and interventions)			
Consider therapeutic care			
- Introduce distraction and/or entertainment			
- Monitor and track behaviour			
- Consider enhanced nursing observation and social interaction (policy)			
- Provide continuity of care-givers to lessen anxiety			
Monitor pain levels and administer prescribed analgesic			
Use FLACC chart			
Elimination – prevent and treat constipation (avoid catheters)			
Avoid unnecessary ward moves			
Environmental control (light level, noise and temperature)			
Ensure patient has access to sensory aids (glasses and hearing aids)			
Encourage mobilisation and activity where possible			
Encourage fluids and diet			
Individualised interventions required:			
- Carer support (open visiting)			
- Advise that recovery often takes weeks/months			
- Give family or carers delirium information leaflet			
- Ensure care reflects the individual's life history, baseline function, preferences and routines (This is me, Forget me not and Hospital Passport, etc.)			
Start date:	Designation and name	Signature	NMC no.

ACTIVITY 5.6: FRANK AND LIZZIE

Frank had been 'off colour' for a few days when he started having episodes where he would become more vague than usual and was agitated and wanting to walk about, particularly at night. He wanted to walk about the bungalow and appeared to be looking for something but couldn't say what he was looking for. Lizzie didn't know if this behaviour was part of Frank's Parkinson's disease but when she tried to prevent him wandering, he would become agitated and shout at her, which was out of character for him.

At 3am, Frank tripped and fell to the floor. Lizzie was unable to help him to his feet so she reluctantly called 999 and the paramedics arranged to transfer Frank to hospital for a thorough check-up. In the Accident and Emergency (A&E) Department, the doctor suspects that Frank has delirium and tells Lizzie that more tests are needed.

How would you respond in this situation?

What are your main areas for action?

Think about how to explain to Lizzie what is happening.

Who else could be available to support Lizzie (daughters or son?)

5.4.2 Client records

Dimond (2005) states that in principle anything that relates to a client within the context of their care can be seen as part of their healthcare records. Nurses are bound by their code to keep clear and accurate records which: "includes but is not limited to patient records. It includes all records that are relevant to your scope of practice" (NMC, 2018a). The NMC Code goes on to say that (see www.nmc.org.uk/standards/code/):

- 10.1 complete records at the time or as soon as possible after an event, recording if the notes are written some time after the event
- 10.2 identify any risks or problems that have arisen and the steps taken to deal with them, so that colleagues who use the records have all the information they need
- 10.3 complete records accurately and without any falsification, taking immediate and appropriate action if you become aware that someone has not kept to these requirements
- 10.4 attribute any entries you make in any paper or electronic records to yourself, making sure they are clearly written, dated and timed, and do not include unnecessary abbreviations, jargon or speculation
- 10.5 take all steps to make sure that records are kept securely
- 10.6 collect, treat and store all data and research findings appropriately.

Furthermore, the NMC states that record-keeping has many important functions and these include a range of clinical, administrative and educational uses and these principles and functions should be related to social care records as well. Good records should:

- help to improve accountability
- show how decisions related to patient care were made
- support the delivery of services

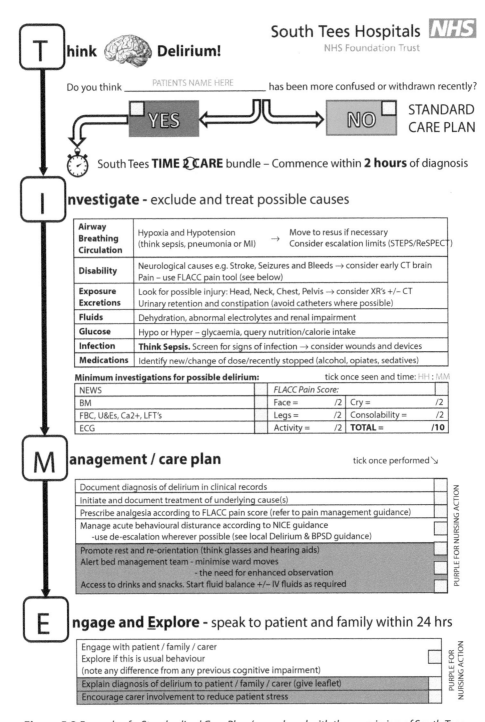

Think Delirium!

South Tees Hospitals **NHS** NHS Foundation Trust

Do you think _____PATIENTS NAME HERE_____ has been more confused or withdrawn recently?

YES ⟸ ⟹ NO STANDARD CARE PLAN

South Tees **TIME 2 CARE** bundle – Commence within **2 hours** of diagnosis

Investigate - exclude and treat possible causes

Airway Breathing Circulation	Hypoxia and Hypotension (think sepsis, pneumonia or MI) →	Move to resus if necessary Consider escalation limits (STEPS/ReSPECT)
Disability	Neurological causes e.g. Stroke, Seizures and Bleeds → consider early CT brain Pain – use FLACC pain tool (see below)	
Exposure Excretions	Look for possible injury: Head, Neck, Chest, Pelvis → consider XR's +/– CT Urinary retention and constipation (avoid catheters where possible)	
Fluids	Dehydration, abnormal electrolytes and renal impairment	
Glucose	Hypo or Hyper – glycaemia, query nutrition/calorie intake	
Infection	**Think Sepsis.** Screen for signs of infection → consider wounds and devices	
Medications	Identify new/change of dose/recently stopped (alcohol, opiates, sedatives)	

Minimum investigations for possible delirium: tick once seen and time: HH : MM

NEWS		FLACC Pain Score:			
BM		Face =	/2	Cry =	/2
FBC, U&Es, Ca2+, LFT's		Legs =	/2	Consolability =	/2
ECG		Activity =	/2	**TOTAL =**	**/10**

Management / care plan   tick once performed ↘

Document diagnosis of delirium in clinical records	
Initiate and document treatment of underlying cause(s)	
Prescribe analgesia according to FLACC pain score (refer to pain management guidance)	
Manage acute behavioural disturance according to NICE guidance -use de-escalation wherever possible (see local Delirium & BPSD guidance)	
Promote rest and re-orientation (think glasses and hearing aids) Alert bed management team - minimise ward moves - the need for enhanced observation Access to drinks and snacks. Start fluid balance +/– IV fluids as required	

PURPLE FOR NURSING ACTION

Engage and **E**xplore - speak to patient and family within 24 hrs

Engage with patient / family / carer Explore if this is usual behaviour (note any difference from any previous cognitive impairment)	
Explain diagnosis of delirium to patient / family / carer (give leaflet)	
Encourage carer involvement to reduce patient stress	

PURPLE FOR NURSING ACTION

Figure 5.2 *Example of a Standardised Care Plan (reproduced with the permission of South Tees Hospitals NHS Foundation Trust).*

- support effective clinical judgements and decisions
- support service user care and communications
- make continuity of care easier
- provide documentary evidence of services delivered
- promote better communication and sharing of information between members of the multi-professional healthcare team
- help to identify risks, enabling early detection of complications
- support clinical audit, research, allocation of resources and performance planning
- help to address complaints or legal processes.

5.4.3 Accountabilities

It is useful to pause and remember that when providing care practitioners are accountable to a number of individuals and organisations:

1. To the individual for whom we are providing care and their family members.
2. To the organisation as employees. Managers can audit care plans to ensure that quality care is being provided.
3. To society which has expectations of care providers.
4. Nurses are professionally accountable to the NMC which sets out the principles of care provision, and tells care recipients what they can expect. If we fail to comply with this, Registered Nurses can be removed from the register and barred from practising.
5. Nurses are legally and ethically accountable to ensure that practitioners work within the jurisdiction of the law for where they work.

Good record-keeping is essential in maintaining those accountabilities.

ACTIVITY 5.7

The principles of good record-keeping apply to all types of records, regardless of how they are held.

List ten types of 'records' that may relate to a single client's care.

Employers usually set the way in which nurses keep records and so different methods for planning care and keeping records are used. It is essential, however, that the principles of good record-keeping are used and that these reflect the core values of individuality and partnership working.

The NMC guidance for record-keeping is now part of the Code (NMC, 2018a) which considers important issues such as:

- ensuring that they are signed and dated
- writing records contemporaneously, ensuring the accuracy and consistency of records
- that records should be written clearly and in such a manner that they cannot be erased, with alterations to dates timed and signed so the author can be identified
- not using jargon or abbreviations
- not using subjective statements which could be offensive or speculative.

One other consideration is that if an episode of care is not recorded then there is no evidence that the care-giving happened. This might have implications for a practitioner who has to attend court, who may not be able to prove that they had complied with their duty to care.

ACTIVITY 5.8: LIZZIE

While providing personal care to Lizzie following her broken ankle, Bernadette, a care worker, notices that the lady has developed a small red patch on her left heel. She is convinced that it was not there when she last visited the lady three days ago. There is nothing noted in the care plan. Bernadette writes the following entry in the care plan: 'Small red patch noted on left heel.'
- How could this episode of record-keeping be improved?
- What might you have recorded here?
- Should this be recorded as a safeguarding issue?

5.4.4 Confidentiality, data and sharing information

One of the issues practitioners need to consider and address at all stages of ASPIRE, but particularly during the record-keeping and planning stages, is the issue of confidentiality. Confidentiality is one of the most important rules of healthcare ethics because confidentiality of information demonstrates respect for the individual (Davis *et al.*, 2006). In healthcare it is about protecting all information about the individual within the Human Rights Act (1998), referring to the right to privacy. The NMC requires practitioners to maintain confidentiality of clients with disclosure only being justified if information is required by law.

ACTIVITY 5.9

Review the NMC Code and see what it states about your professional duty to protect confidentiality.

The sharing of information across health and social care supports multidisciplinary assessment and planning and can lead to individuals getting the support that underpins their independence and the outcomes they want for their lives by enabling choice. If information collected at different sources can be drawn together it can save time and also address practical issues such as individuals needing to repeat information to a number of different professionals. The proliferation of IT over the last two decades has therefore brought new opportunities and new challenges to keeping records.

Practitioners need to be fully aware of the legal requirements and guidance regarding confidentiality and ensure practice is in line with national and local policies when keeping and storing records. Consideration should be given to any information that can identify a person in your care as it must not be used or disclosed for purposes other than health and social care without the individual's explicit consent. The exception to this is that you can release this information if the law requires it, or where there is a wider public interest, such as a public health issue like an outbreak of diarrhoea and vomiting in a care home.

The General Data Protection Regulation (GDPR) came into effect in May 2018 and is designed to allow individuals to have more control about how their data is collected, stored and used. It essentially protects individuals by ensuring personal data can only be used if consent is given. The right to access of that data belongs to the individual. Any organisation breaching the rules is subject to very large fines. This has huge implications for the sharing of information about individuals and all healthcare employers will have put policies in place to ensure they are compliant. This will include all employees having mandatory training and makes the part of the Code that states "take all steps to make sure that all records are kept securely" (NMC, 2018a) hold a much more stringent legal imperative.

Thus, while the opportunity of a national IT network, with the possibility of sharing records between professionals and across professions and services is valuable, it is important to consider the security of IT systems. Security measures such as Smartcards or passwords to access information systems must not be shared or systems left open to access when you have finished using them, in order to prevent unauthorised individuals having access to confidential information.

However, computer-held records do offer a number of advantages in addition to information sharing:
- the ability to audit care
- the ability to use templates and standardised planning to improve the approach to care planning and record-keeping
- the ability to use data to audit records.

The ability to use data to audit records does, however, highlight the importance of data quality. The quality of information from systems is only as good as the information that goes into a system. Shared standards, common coding and an agreement across professional groups not to replicate data is crucial to its success.

It is also important to remember that people have the legal right to ask to see their own health records and different public sector organisations will have local policies, which you must be aware of; organisations employing health and social care staff will have policy and guidelines to address this need.

ACTIVITY 5.10

Find your local policy on record-keeping and sharing, and your Trust's policy on GDPR.

List the key principles of the policy.

What does the policy say in relation to sharing information?

What situations might require information being shared with other agencies?

Check you have completed the mandatory GDPR training.

Requests to withhold information must be respected unless withholding such information would cause serious harm to that person or others; under common law, you are allowed to disclose information if it will help to prevent, detect, investigate or punish serious crime or if it will prevent abuse or serious harm to others.

Finally, it is important that confidentiality is applied to all areas of practice. It is essential that discussions concerning the people in your care are not conducted in places where you might be overheard. This applies to areas in your place of work just as it does outside, for example on the bus on the way home! It is equally important that records, either on paper or on computer screens, are not left or placed where they might be seen by unauthorised staff or members of the public. You should not access the records of any person, or their family, to find out personal information that is not relevant to their care.

5.5 The practicalities of care planning

We have seen that care planning can be very complex and relies on the interpersonal skills of the professional working with the patient in order to hear and understand what their wants and needs are. It also involves working within the therapeutic relationship to ensure partnership is achieved (see *Chapter 4*).

A further consideration is the practical one of resources. It is an imperative part of the planning stage of ASPIRE to plan care based on local and national guidance and financial resources. This should be based on current evidence and consideration of the financial resources available to the services in question. Evidence-based interventions will be discussed in more detail in *Chapter 6*.

ACTIVITY 5.11

Think back to Scott, Frank and Lizzie's grandson.

Referring to national guidance on the treatment of obesity and researching through the internet, identify the estimated cost of obesity to the UK, in terms of morbidity and associated medical and social conditions, e.g. lost working days. Considering these costs, do you think that addressing obesity should be a priority for services? Are there any evidence-based (and therefore cost-effective) treatments or interventions for obesity?

CHAPTER SUMMARY

Building on the assessment chapter, *Chapter 5* has examined the nature of planning care and support, looking at both goal setting and the use of SMART objectives and MACROS and how this is important within a phased approach to planning the care process. Partnership working within the multidisciplinary team and through collaborative working with service users and carers has been explored within the context of a resource-constrained service. We have demonstrated the importance of ensuring that a plan or intervention is realistic, explicit, evidence-based, prioritised, involved and goal-centred (REEPIG) in order to deliver the intended outcomes. The importance of keeping accurate written records and confidentiality has been discussed. The role of information technology in health and social care has been considered, as well as the implications of the increased use of IT within health and social care. Finally, we have discussed the fact that when providing care, practitioners are accountable to a number of individuals and organisations and good record-keeping is essential to this.

Reflection

Identify at least three things that you have learned from this chapter.	1. ....
	2. ....
	3. ....
How do you plan to use this knowledge within clinical practice?	1. ....
	2. ....
	3. ....
How will you evaluate the effectiveness of your plan?	1. ....
	2. ....
	3. ....
What further knowledge and evidence do you need?	1. ....
	2. ....
	3. ....

FURTHER READING

Cuthbert, S. and Quallington, J. (2017) *Values and Ethics for Care Practice*. Banbury: Lantern Publishing.

Values and ethics are integral to the provision, practice and delivery of patient-centred health and social care. This book, which is an expanded and updated version of the 2008 title *Values for Care Practice*, introduces readers to these concepts and helps them understand how they can apply them to become compassionate care professionals.

The patient perspective and patient voice are seen and heard throughout the book. Readers are encouraged to reflect on their personal values and on those underpinning health and social care work and to understand how values and ethics are articulated in the latest Codes of Practice. The text uses activities and case studies to enable readers to apply theory in their practice.

This book will help readers to understand why good caring is more than merely a practical intervention; it also requires a personal investment and quality of character that involves genuine concern and respect for others.

Marquis, B. and Huston, C. (2017) *Leadership Roles and Management Functions in Nursing: theory and application*, 9th edition. London: Lippincott.

Now in its ninth edition, this foremost leadership and management text incorporates application with theory and emphasises critical thinking, problem-solving and decision-making. More than 280 learning exercises promote critical thinking and interactive discussion. Case studies cover a variety of settings, including acute care, ambulatory care, long-term care and community health. The book addresses timely issues such as leadership development, staffing, delegation, ethics and law, organisational, political and personal power, management and technology, and more. Web links and learning exercises appear in each chapter.

National Involvement Standards (2015) *Involvement for Influence*. Available at: www.nationalvoices.org.uk/sites/default/files/public/4pinationalinvolvement standardsfullreport20152.pdf (accessed 4 June 2019)

This report sets out its main tasks as developing national involvement standards in mental health and hardwiring involvement into the planning, delivery and evaluation of mental health services. The key themes of equalising power, recognising diversity and commitment to genuine change are explored.

Chapter 6
Implementation

LEARNING OUTCOMES

This chapter covers the following key issues:

- The nature of intervention in health and social care

- Types of healthcare intervention

- Evidence-based interventions

- Working in partnership to enable intervention activity

- Advocacy

By the end of this chapter you should be able to:

- ensure that the care you provide in the implementation phase of the care process is holistic and person-centred

- articulate the rationale for undertaking types of interventions in healthcare

- discuss the importance of working in partnership to implement care

- identify the importance of culturally appropriate caring

- reflect on what role healthcare practitioners have in advocacy.

While many elements of the NMC platforms that make up the standards of proficiency for registered nurses are covered, this chapter has particular reference to (NMC, 2018b):

- Platform 1: Being an accountable professional

- Platform 4: Providing and evaluating care

For further detailed mapping please see *Appendix 1* – Detailed mapping to *Future Nurse: standards of proficiency for registered nurses*.

6.1 **Introduction**

Implementation is the third phase of the cycle of ASPIRE (*Figure 6.1*).

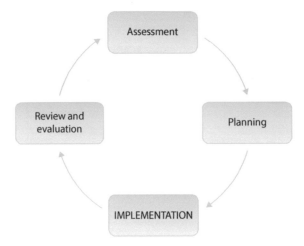

Figure 6.1 *Implementation, the third phase of the ASPIRE cycle.*

The implementation phase of the care process is concerned with the provision of care and so the implementation of the care plan. There are three key issues that need to be considered when discussing intervention:
1. How the care will be implemented
2. The nature of the intervention
3. How to involve the patient and carer.

We will look at each of these in turn, but it is important to bear in mind that these aspects are all interconnected.

6.2 **Person-centred care**

We live in a diverse society, with a plurality of beliefs between individuals, families and members of social groups. Person-centred practice is care that recognises the circumstances, concerns, goals, beliefs and cultures of the individual, their family and friends. Each individual is unique and has unique needs, so it is important to acknowledge the significance of spiritual, emotional and religious support.

> *Care is delivered in a sensitive, person-centred way that takes account of the circumstances, wishes and priorities of the individual, their family and friends.* *End of Life Care Strategy*, available at https://assets.publishing.service.gov.uk/government/uploads/system/uploads/attachment_data/file/136431/End_of_life_strategy.pdf

6.2.1 Holistic care

The term 'holistic' comes from the word 'whole' and holistic care usually refers to considering the whole person as opposed to caring for 'the appendectomy in bed 4'.

It is recognised that aspects such as biology, psychology and emotional wellbeing, mental health and social dimensions impact upon a person's ability to care for themselves. People live with spiritual beliefs and in environments that impact on health (see also *Chapter 1*).

There are a number of different ways and processes of delivering care that can make a difference to a person's life and address their needs. Within a holistic framework of care, interventions can focus on making a difference in the physical, psychological, social, spiritual and/or environmental domains of a person's life. Maslow's (1962) hierarchy of needs (*Figure 6.2*) is a useful framework to demonstrate the levels of need that care interventions might focus on to improve a care recipient's health and social wellbeing.

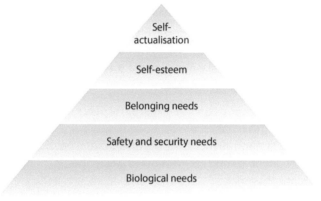

Figure 6.2 *Maslow's (1962) hierarchy of needs.*

ACTIVITY 6.1: FRANK

Think back to the case study about Lizzie and Frank.

Can you identify Frank's needs using Maslow's hierarchy of needs?

Biological needs are fundamental to a person's wellbeing and capacity to achieve their maximum potential within a holistic concept of self. Interventions to address biological needs are sometimes referred to as basic care (Henderson, 1960). However, this can be misleading, as the term 'basic' can be misconstrued as menial. The provision of good-quality and timely interventions to address biological needs is a highly skilled activity, involving the use of a range of psychomotor and interpersonal skills to provide care in an individualised manner that respects the care recipient's dignity and self-worth.

The fundamental aspects of caring include being able to recognise which need is a priority. For example, in a cardiac arrest situation, the patient does not require you to consider their emotional wellbeing; the biological need is the priority. But when a patient is fit for discharge and preparing to be discharged from hospital to a care home, the routine daily temperature recording is less likely to be important than their emotional care.

6.2.2 Dignity and respect

The right to be treated with dignity and respect is a fundamental human right and is enshrined in the Human Rights Act (1998). In November 2006, the Dignity in Care Campaign in health and social care was launched. The campaign has been updated with new guidance published in 2013 but the principle remains (Department of Health, 2006):

> High quality health and social care services should be delivered in a person-centred way that respects the dignity of the individual receiving them.

> Every breach of human dignity not only affects the individual victim, but also society as a whole, by raising the question of how we choose to live (and die) and relate to each other. It thereby calls into question the state's role in protecting our dignity.
>
> (Dupré, 2011)

The Royal College of Nursing also supports this notion. It argues that when dignity is absent from care, people feel devalued, lacking control and comfort. They may also lack confidence, be unable to make decisions for themselves, and feel humiliated, embarrassed and ashamed.

Providing dignity in care centres on three integral aspects: respect, compassion and sensitivity. In practice, this means:

- **Respecting** patients' and clients' diversity and cultural needs; their privacy – including protecting it as much as possible in large, open-plan hospital wards; and the decisions they make.
- Being **compassionate** when a patient or client and/or their relatives need emotional support, rather than just delivering technical nursing care.
- Demonstrating **sensitivity** to patients' and clients' needs, ensuring their comfort.

Patients and clients can also experience dignity – or its absence – in what they wear, such as gowns, and in the physical environment where treatment takes place. For example, according to the RCN's Dignity Campaign (www.dignityincare.org.uk/Resources/Type/RCN-Dignity-Campaign):

- facilities such as toilets should be well maintained and cleaned regularly
- curtains between beds should close properly to offer some measure of privacy
- toilet doors should be closed when in use
- bays in wards should be single-sex
- gowns should be designed and made in a way that allows them to be fastened properly to avoid accidental exposure
- privacy should be provided for private conversations, intimate care and personal activities, such as going to the toilet.

Older people and dignity

A number of areas where care interventions did not treat older people with dignity have been identified by the Care Quality Commission (Department of Health, 2008b, Regulation 10):

- Patients were addressed in an inappropriate manner or spoken about as if they were not there.

- People were not given information or did not have their consent sought or wishes considered.
- People were left in soiled clothes or exposed in an embarrassing manner.
- Appropriate food or help with eating was not given.
- People were placed in mixed-sex accommodation.

It is therefore imperative that health and social care practitioners are aware of the impact of care on individuals and build up a relationship of trust so that interventions can be carried out in a sensitive and competent manner, according to the service user's wishes and best interests (see discussion of malignant social psychology in *Section 2.4*).

6.2.3 Privileged access

It is important to remember to treat people with dignity in all encounters, but this is particularly important in areas of physical and emotional privileged access. Privileged access in relation to healthcare refers to the fact that healthcare professionals are legitimately able to touch people in intimate areas (with consent) and conduct invasive procedures (such as rectal examination). In addition, healthcare professionals have privileged access in interactions with relative strangers as they can legitimately ask intimate questions in the assessment of needs.

ACTIVITY 6.2

Think about a practice encounter that you have been in recently.
- List the interventions that you engaged in.
- In what ways did you have privileged access to the individual?

6.2.4 Culturally relevant and appropriate care

Care is organised around the needs and circumstances of the individual, and is delivered in a co-ordinated manner across services. It is delivered in a way that demonstrates respect for the individual, their family and friends, maintaining their dignity at all times. Workers are sensitive to circumstances, and their changing nature, and care is delivered accordingly.
End of Life Care Strategy, available at https://assets.publishing.service.gov.uk/government/uploads/system/uploads/attachment_data/file/136431/End_of_life_strategy.pdf

The UK today is a multicultural, multi-ethnic and multiple-language society and so the provision of culturally appropriate and relevant care interventions is a fundamental issue for health and social care professionals. Culture is made up of beliefs, values and ideas about what is right and what is wrong and these guide a person's behaviours or customs (Richardson, 2009). It is important that care-givers explore the ways in which they can provide appropriate care to individuals, whose ethnic, cultural and race backgrounds are different to their own. Professional codes of conduct and organisational policies and guidelines will make it very clear to health and social care staff that ignorance of cultural needs or prejudicial attitudes are not acceptable.

Culture, ethnicity and race

Culture is characterised by a person's upbringing and choices, which lead to behaviours and attitudes that can be changed, for example by adapting to different cultures. Ethnicity is characterised as a sense of belonging and group identity determined by group pressures and psychological need. Race is characterised by physical appearance and genetic history, which can be argued to be as irrelevant as hair or eye colour (Richardson, 2009).

ACTIVITY 6.3

Think of your own ethnic/cultural background.

What differences of behaviour or attitudes can you list within your own ethnic or cultural 'group'?

Think about religion, sexual orientation, diet.

Think about your parents or grandparents. How is your behaviour culturally different from previous generations?

It is, however, also important for healthcare practitioners to acknowledge that it is not enough simply to understand the care recipient's culture but also to have an awareness of the impact of their own cultural norms on their care-giving by developing their knowledge of self through reflection (*Table 6.1*). This will help the individual to recognise and address feelings about 'difference' that they may not even have recognised before but which may have played a part in subconscious behaviours that challenge an individual's ability to achieve unconditional acceptance. If left unaddressed this can lead to discrimination (Richardson, 2009). For example, it might be your family custom to use the expression 'God bless you' or suggest that 'I will pray for you', but other people could take offence at these phrases, despite your intention to be kind.

Table 6.1 *Essential elements of culturally competent care (taken from ACECQA: https://wehearyou.acecqa.gov.au/2014/07/10/what-does-it-mean-to-be-culturally-competent/)*

Educators who respect diversity and are culturally competent:
- have an understanding of, and honour, the histories, cultures, languages, traditions, child rearing practices
- value different capacities and abilities
- respect differences in families' home lives
- recognise that diversity contributes to the richness of society and provides a valid evidence base about ways of knowing
- demonstrate an ongoing commitment to developing cultural competence in a two-way process with families and communities
- teach, role-model and encourage cultural competence in children, recognising that this is crucial to ensuring children have a sense of strong cultural identity and belonging
- engage in ongoing reflection relating to their cultural competence and how they build cultural competence.

There are many situations within the care encounter where cultural differences impact and these could include (Hayes and Llewellyn, 2008, p. 204):

- personal space (proximity of where you stand)
- eye contact (direct or non-direct eye contact)
- physical contact (gender and modesty)
- diet (foods and products containing food derivatives).

While paying attention to cultural issues in care is important, it is also essential to acknowledge that by identifying a care recipient as belonging to a cultural minority group may be useful, as you are identifying beliefs, values and customs, such an emphasis on group can also be problematic (Richardson, 2009). It is important to avoid making stereotypes or assumptions about a person's culture based on your perceptions of the group they belong to rather than asking them themselves. Individuality and valuing the individual remains the principle here. The best way to check out what is appropriate is to ask the person.

6.3 Types of intervention

Interventions may be designed to focus primarily on a specific task, although assessment of need should have been conducted within a holistic framework. Thus, interventions may be based on the planned achievement of certain goals, or they may be implemented to address a specific crisis or event, such as the cardiac arrest or discharge planning.

6.3.1 Task-centred interventions

Task allocation as a system of intervention in nursing practice has been widely criticised, as it leads to a fragmentation of care and a lack of focus on the holistic care of the individual. Menzies (1960) also argues that the system of task allocation prevented nurses from becoming too involved with the patient and helped them to retain a social distance and protect themselves from emotional engagement. It could also be argued that it is less satisfying for the practitioner, who engages in a series of repetitive tasks rather than utilising a range of skills and knowledge to achieve holistic care. As stated previously, the provision of care is an interpersonal activity, and the focus on the division of labour and the allocation of tasks militates against person-centred and individualised care, reducing the care task to a sort of assembly line activity, with a focus on outcome at the expense of quality and process.

However, there may be times or occasions where task allocation is a highly efficient way to manage to deliver a minimum standard of safe care, for a limited period of time; for example, sudden staff shortages or evacuating a ward in a fire situation.

ACTIVITY 6.4: LIZZIE

Lizzie has been feeling tired lately and her GP would like her to have blood tests and a chest X-ray. She gives Lizzie two request cards to take to the hospital outpatient department for the blood test and chest X-ray. When Lizzie arrives, she speaks to the receptionist and explains why she is there. She is asked to wait in seating area A. After a few minutes, the phlebotomist calls Lizzie to follow her to a clinical room to take her blood samples. Lizzie is then asked to return to seating area B. Lizzie has another short wait until a receptionist from X-ray calls Lizzie and takes her to the changing area and asks Lizzie to undress and wear the hospital gown and then wait in area F. The radiologist eventually calls Lizzie and takes her to the X-ray room to have her X-ray. When the X-ray is checked, Lizzie is told she can go home.

How might you measure the efficiency of the experience for Lizzie?

How person-centred is this approach?

What skills would the practitioners need to demonstrate to show that they care?

6.3.2 Crisis intervention

Crisis intervention approaches are also often used in healthcare work. They have their roots in developmental psychology and cognitive behavioural psychology, but in reality, draw on a range of different theoretical perspectives (McGinnis, 2009). Often when people engage with healthcare services, they are experiencing some sort of crisis (whether it is interpersonal, physical, emotional, spiritual or social or a combination).

Imagine that you were to have a stroke today. How would that impact on your immediate biological needs, then subsequently, what would be the impact on your emotional and spiritual needs? At some point in the future, you would also have to consider your financial needs if you could not return to work.

Stress

Stress is an important concept to consider here, and how we help people to manage the stressors that they are experiencing and work with their own resilience and coping strategies. We all experience stress throughout our lives and find ways to manage this stress. Some degree of stress is helpful, because it motivates us to do things (eustress). When stress becomes unmanageable (distress), either because of the unusual nature of it (as in physical crisis) or because of severity, duration or a multiplicity of stressors, then a person may require intervention from healthcare practitioners.

ACTIVITY 6.5

Think about a recent stressful event that you experienced (this might be something like a new social encounter or engaging with a new and unfamiliar task).

How did the stress make you feel?

How did you manage the stress and cope with the situation?

What skills did you draw on from your coping in previous stressful encounters?

Safeguarding vulnerable individuals is an important aspect of crisis intervention. This might sometimes involve invoking safeguarding procedures in order to ensure that they are protected from abusive or neglectful environments. Procedures and policies for intervention where there is suspected or alleged abuse or neglect are set out in statute in The Children Act for children and in the Safeguarding Adults guidance for vulnerable adults (see www.tsab.org.uk/ for up-to-date guidance).

6.3.3 Continual intervention

Continual interventions are those interventions that help to determine a course of action and maintain the safety of the patient over a period of time. This may also require continual assessment, planning and evaluation, as can be seen from the skills that are required.

Skills needed for continual intervention

1. **Observation** – practitioners are constantly observing the people they work with for changes in their condition. This might include observation of:
   - vital signs (temperature, heart rate, respirations, oxygen saturations, blood pressure)
   - appearance (e.g. skin colour – pallor or flushed)
   - non-verbal communications (pain, anxiety, limb weakness)
   - responses to medication (improvements and side-effects)
   - signs of risk and the need for protection and safeguarding; in the Laming Report (Lord Laming, 2009) following the death of Baby P (Peter Connelly), professionals were criticised for failing to observe or interpret signs of abuse and neglect.
2. **Inspection** – there is a clear role for practitioners to examine service users for any changes in their condition. This could include, for example:
   - the inspection of a wound or pressure sore to detect any improvements or deteriorations (see also *Chapter 7*).
3. **Monitoring** – this involves checking on a regular basis and is an effective intervention in preventative practice. For example, dentists monitor the condition of teeth through regular check-ups, while health visitors and school nurses monitor child growth and development. Individuals may also self-monitor: for example, a person with diabetes may monitor their blood glucose level or urinary glucose on a regular basis, while someone on a reducing diet may weigh themselves on a weekly basis. Self-monitoring and self-evaluation are fundamental to changes in healthcare practice, which emphasise person-centred care and the notion of the service user as the expert in their own care as identified within the Department of Health's Expert Patient Programme (Department of Health, 2008c).
4. **Listening** – a number of diagnostic tools can be used to listen for signs and changes in conditions:
   - Stethoscopes (listen to chest for signs of infection)
   - Doppler (a form of ultrasound to listen for pedal pulses)
   - Sonicaid (to listen for the baby's heartbeat in the uterus).

The practitioner's own listening skills are also important and can be used to listen for non-verbalised signs. For example, a practitioner may be able to pick up on anxiety, pain and suffering through listening to changes in the voice, and practitioners are increasingly encouraged through models of professional practice to listen to what the service users and carers have to say (see also *Chapter 2*).

6.3.4 Therapeutic interventions

Therapeutic interventions are those interventions that maintain the strengths and coping abilities of the service user and carer, as well as treating problems. Therapeutic interventions involve a range of helping skills, and can be used for a variety of reasons:

- meeting fundamental needs
- helping people to develop their own self-care skills
- assisting with activities of daily living and problem-solving.

Therapeutic interventions can also be used to demonstrate caring and to provide relaxation and improve self-esteem. Tutton (1991), for example, identifies touch as a way of communicating care and wellbeing. In this sense, touch can convey messages of acceptance and trust and can therefore be therapeutic. In addition, Routasalo and Isola (1998) conclude that touch can be therapeutic when it has a calming and comforting effect on a service user.

ACTIVITY 6.6

Consider times when you have maybe held a patient's hand to comfort them.

What impact did this have?

(See also discussion of touch in *Chapter 2*)

Health education and health promotion are also important therapeutic interventions, and reflect the contemporary policy agenda in relation to prevention of disease and illness. Public health initiatives, which consist of delivering health promotion programmes, can be key interventions enabling the prevention of disease, disability or illness and healthcare practitioners are in a key position to deliver this type of intervention (Coverdale, 2009). Health promotion is, on the one hand, the prevention and control of premature death and disease and, on the other, the promotion of wellbeing and control over health. This can be achieved through both empowering and enabling individuals, which helps to make healthy choices easier (Tones and Green, 2004).

Intervention can take place at an individual level, where service users are enabled to understand their disease or disability better through access to information, education or services or when they are enabled to explore the ways in which they can cope with their circumstance by one-to-one intervention with a single practitioner.

Intervention can also take place at population level. This may include a host of health-promoting campaigns such as the child immunisation programme or media campaigns delivering health messages such as the Change4Life campaign and involve building health promotion activities into a care plan for an individual, e.g. quit smoking interventions.

ACTIVITY 6.7

Michelle is a 25-year-old woman with a learning disability who lives with her parents. You have been providing support to Michelle and her family for some time. Her mother rings you to tell you that Michelle has started a sexual relationship and 'it has to stop'. She is concerned that Michelle is being 'taken advantage of' and that her boyfriend is abusive towards her. She says that her daughter should not be allowed to have a sexual relationship.

To find out more, you speak to a worker at the day centre Michelle attends. The worker informs you that they are aware of the sexual relationship she is having. However, they do not feel comfortable speaking to Michelle about this and don't think this is something that they should deal with. The worker is not clear whether Michelle is being abused in any way.

You arrange to see Michelle. Michelle becomes distressed when you broach the subject of her new relationship. She does not seem clear about sexual protection issues. You notice that she has a large bruise on her arm. When you ask Michelle about this, she says she tripped over on the stairs.

How would you assess Michelle's needs and what types of interventions would your plan include?

Issues that you might consider:
- Investigative skills to assess whether abuse is taking place
- Interventions to safeguard Michelle if abuse is taking place
- Interventions to assess capacity
- Information about alternative decisions
- Health education/health promotion about safe sex (unwanted pregnancy/sexually transmitted diseases)
- Support for Michelle to make decisions if she has capacity
- Support for Michelle's parents
- Education and training for day centre staff
- Communication skills to develop a relationship of trust with Michelle and her parents
- Health education/health promotion about safe sex and consensual sex for Michelle's boyfriend.

Interventions therefore can be performed in a variety of ways, depending on the intended outcome. Contemporary policy imperatives stress the importance of early intervention and interventions aimed at preventing problems occurring (Bate, 2017). Effective interventions can then take a number of forms and it is important that the appropriate intervention is used to address the needs as identified in the assessment process and to achieve the specific aims of the care plan. It is also important that interventions have a sound evidence base.

6.4 Evidence-based practice

Interventions should be based on sound theoretical knowledge. There is a plethora of definitions of evidence-based practice (EBP), from those that feel distinctly medical to those involving professional judgement of some kind, to those recognising the implicit nature of involving the individual patient or care recipient involved. There are also definitions that recognise the importance of the effective use of resources and that EBP has to be actively pursued and managed (*Table 6.2*).

Table 6.2 *Definitions of evidence-based practice*

Context or 'feel'	Definitions
EBP as distinctly medical	Evidence-based medicine is the use of mathematical estimates of the risk of benefit and harm, derived from high quality research on population samples, to inform clinical decision-making in the diagnosis, investigation or management of individual service users. (Greenhalgh, 2000)
EBP as involving professional judgement of some kind	The conscientious, explicit and judicious use of current best evidence in making decisions about the care of individual service users. The practice of evidence-based medicine means integrating individual clinical expertise with the best available external clinical evidence from systematic research. (Sackett *et al.*, 1996)
EBP as recognising the implicit nature of involving the individual patient or care recipient	Evidence-based clinical practice is an approach to decision-making in which the clinician uses the best evidence available, in consultation with the patient, to decide upon the option which suits that patient best. (Muir Gray, 1997)
EBP as effective use of resources	The process of systematically finding, appraising and using contemporaneous research findings as a basis for clinical decisions. It aims to eliminate the use of expensive, ineffective and dangerous medical decision-making. (Rosenberg and Donald, 1995)
But also that it has to be actively pursued and managed:	Evidence-based practice has grown out of the desire by practitioners and managers that services that are provided are based on the best research evidence available. (Law, 2000)

Sackett *et al.*'s definition (2000) that EBP can be defined as "the integration of best research evidence with expertise and patient (or client) values" incorporates three principles of practice which are required to optimise clinical (and non-clinical) outcomes but also importantly quality of life:

- relevant research
- the ability of the practitioner to use clinical (and non-clinical) skills and past experiences to support each individual person's unique health state, their individual risks and benefits to potential interventions and their personal values and expectations
- the uniqueness, concerns and preferences that each patient brings which must be integrated into care decisions.

Sackett *et al.* (2000) argue that EBP comprises five steps (*Figure 6.3*):

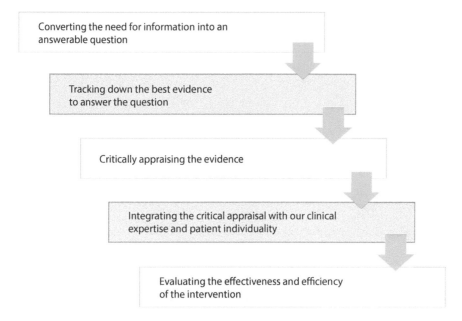

Figure 6.3 *Five Steps of EBP (adapted from Sackett* et al., *2000).*

It is important to acknowledge that EBP is the responsibility of all professionals as colleagues of all skill mixes and experience can provide new evidence to influence practice. It is in the best interest of patients/clients to continuously question what we know and do and to change practices where there is an indication that they can be improved on. EBP is about:

- doing what works (does more good than harm)
- doing what is (or is most) effective
- doing what works best (does *most* good)
- what is most cost-effective (does most good per £ spent)
- doing what is most efficient (timely)
- doing what raises patient/client 'satisfaction'.

However, it is also important to acknowledge that there is not an evidence base for all practice and this is where the concept of best practice fits in. Best practice refers to practice where the technique, method, process, activity and intervention is agreed to be the most efficient (least amount of effort) and effective (best results) way of accomplishing a task, based on the experience and agreement of expert practitioners.

6.5 Patient and carer involvement

Person-centred care suggests patients and their carers should be involved in decisions about their care and the interventions that are proposed by professionals to support them. Shared decision-making is a process by which individuals are supported by health professionals to make decisions about how they are cared for.

ACTIVITY 6.8: FRANK

Frank has been referred to see the Parkinson's disease specialist nurse to see whether he can make any recommendations to enhance Frank's quality of life. After a long discussion, the nurse suggests that Frank might be eligible to take part in a clinical trial that is testing a new medical intervention. The trial would involve Frank having a blood test every week at the GP surgery on a Sunday. Frank and Lizzie consider the involvement but the weekly blood test would interfere with them attending the Salvation Army church service. They want to decline the invitation but feel a bit awkward as the nurse is 'a lovely young man'.

How can they be supported to make the decision that is right for them?

What skills would the practitioners need to demonstrate to show that they care?

6.5.1 Skills for intervention

Beresford (2007) identified the key elements that service users value in their relationships with professionals, and concluded that a social approach to intervention is seen as particularly beneficial, stressing the importance of the interrelationship and the attributes of:

- warmth
- respect
- a non-judgemental approach
- listening
- treating people with equality
- trustworthiness
- an open and honest approach
- reliability
- good communication skills.

Service users value practitioners who give them time to sort things out for themselves and who provide support for them to work out their own agendas (Beresford, 2007).

6.5.2 Advocacy

Advocacy is one form of intervention that involves the patient and carer. Advocacy can be defined as individual and group actions to affect change by writing and/or speaking in support of an issue outside of one's immediate group (Winkleby *et al.*, 2004). Advocacy serves as a mechanism to enable people to take control over their own lives. In a study of people with learning disabilities, Thomas and Woods (2003) demonstrate how advocacy services were used to enable participation and social inclusion.

The overarching principle of advocacy is that each person has a value, the capacity to grow and develop and (importantly) to participate. It fits within the context of 'society', which gives rise to human and legal rights and the concept of citizenship. The legal definition of citizenship is the status of a person recognised under the custom or law as a legal member of a sovereign state or belonging to a nation, but it also refers to a person's obligation to contribute to the society or community in which they live or indeed that community's responsibility to protect their individual citizens.

In nursing, advocacy is often seen when the nurse acts as an advocate for the vulnerable, representing their best interests; for example, in challenging poor practice.

ACTIVITY 6.9

Consider your professional group.

How does your employer legislate to ensure the rights of your service users are protected in this way?

The role of the health and social care practitioner in advocacy

For individuals who are disempowered through their circumstances of ill health or their social care needs, there may be a need for health and social care practitioners to intervene on their behalf and advocate or arrange for appropriate advocacy for them. In the NMC Code it is stated that nurses must "act as an advocate for the vulnerable, challenging poor practice and discriminatory attitudes and behaviour relating to their care" (NMC, 2018a).

It may be a question of a practitioner questioning a circumstance and taking a series of actions or steps that lead the circumstance towards what should be. Put simply, taking actions to change the "what is" into a "what should be". Advocacy, however, does not always take place on an individual level as these five principle types of advocacy show (Rapaport *et al.*, 2005):

- Legal advocacy – broad range of methods and strategies using statutory frameworks and legislation (e.g. Human Rights Act 1988).

- Class advocacy – this can be collective action, corporate or group action, and involves groups working together to promote the interests of the group, e.g. MIND, Age UK, the MS Society. Such groups can function in many ways, such as, for example, giving a voice to (misrepresented) citizen interests; mobilising citizens to participate in the democratic process; assisting in the development of better public policy through lobbying.
- Self-advocacy – process of empowerment (see *Chapter 8*) used to encourage vulnerable and marginalised people to have a voice and to advocate for their own needs. This type of advocacy is central to anti-oppressive practice and fits with interventions designed to give people skills and opportunities to develop knowledge and confidence. It is fundamental to person-centred care and self-directed support.
- Peer advocacy – people with similar experiences speak on behalf of others – examples would be local support projects and groups.
- Citizen advocacy – vulnerable people or people with needs are linked to a volunteer who would advocate on their behalf (e.g. befriending services for older people).

One of the tensions for health and social care practitioners is being able to advocate for service users, where resource constraints and other pressures may conflict with this role. There is no easy answer to this ethical dilemma. One way to address this is to signpost service users and carers to local advocacy services, so that they can access appropriate support. Thus an awareness of the relevant services is an important tool in managing the ethical dilemmas that arise in a resource-constrained care environment (McDonald, 2006).

CHAPTER SUMMARY

By introducing intervention within the ASPIRE framework of the care process, this chapter has considered the nature and types of intervention in health and social care, discussing the reasons and rationale for undertaking specific interventions. The importance of using evidence-based interventions has been explored in terms of both cost-effectiveness and efficiency. Building on *Chapter 5* it has re-emphasised the importance of working in partnership in order to enable intervention activity and has considered the role of advocacy for health and social care practitioners.

Reflection

Identify at least three things that you have learned from this chapter.

1. ....
   ....
2. ....
   ....
3. ....
   ....

How do you plan to use this
knowledge within clinical practice?

1. ....

....

2. ....

....

3. ....

....

How will you evaluate the
effectiveness of your plan?

1. ....

....

2. ....

....

3. ....

....

What further knowledge and
evidence do you need?

1. ....

....

2. ....

....

3. ....

....

FURTHER READING

Aveyard, H. and Sharp, P. (2017) *A Beginner's Guide to Evidence Based Practice in Health and Social Care*, 3rd edition. London: Open University Press.

This book is for anyone who has ever wondered what evidence-based practice is or how to relate it to practice. Using everyday language, this book provides a step-by-step guide to what we mean by evidence-based practice and how to apply it. It also:

- provides an easy-to-follow guide to searching for evidence
- explains how to work out if the evidence is relevant or not
- explores how evidence can be applied in the practice setting
- outlines how evidence can be incorporated into your academic writing.

Donnelly, E., Parkinson, T. and Williams, B. (2009) *Understanding and Helping People in Crisis*. Exeter: Reflect Press.

This book is a user-friendly and accessible guide for all those who support people who are experiencing personal crisis. Aimed at both students and practitioners, it introduces the reader to the concept of crisis, touching upon global perspectives, local emergencies and personal experiences. Also, as a means of illustrating common experiences, the book presents a new model of crisis. It reviews personal narratives that reflect a range of common crises encountered in ordinary lives. The narratives and case studies reviewed identify gender and cultural influences alongside family, home and relationships as well as the impact that outside agencies, economics and occupation have on an individual at a time of crisis. It explores crisis theory – psychoanalytical theories, mental health, coping mechanisms and a transactional analysis perspective are explored, as well as cognitive and behavioural understandings of what happens to individuals when a crisis situation occurs – and offers an overview of crisis interventions. This discussion is enhanced through the detail of practical skills that have proved to be helpful in supporting people in crisis. Finally, it reviews the potential outcomes for crisis. Positive and negative crisis resolutions, potential for recovery and change are explored and personal narratives are revisited. The final section includes detail regarding the more serious outcomes of crisis including post-traumatic stress disorder, mental illness and the potential for suicide.

Heaslip, V. and Lindsay, B. (2019) *Research and Evidence-Based Practice.* Banbury: Lantern Publishing.

This accessible and easy-to-read text enables students to understand what research is and how it can provide evidence for practice. It uses clear explanations, key case studies, questions and activities to explore the principles of research needed for students to develop their own evidence-based practice. It covers areas such as why research is carried out and why it matters, and gives thorough guidance on how to search and review the literature in order to evaluate the quality of research. It explores how research projects are designed and participants recruited, how data is collected and analysed, and how research findings are communicated. It also covers important areas related to the cost and funding of research, ethics, and how to review evidence and use it to improve the quality of care. For the student, it has a practical and applied approach that enables the development of ways to both demonstrate the understanding of research and evidence, and to develop and promote best practice in health and social care.

Chapter 7
Review and evaluation

LEARNING OUTCOMES

This chapter covers the following key issues:

- Evaluation and review of health and social care
- Quality drivers for contemporary health and social care policy
- Professionalism and professional standards
- The implementation of evidence-based practice into everyday working practice
- Benchmarking
- Critical incident analysis and reflective practice
- Theory and models of quality assurance
- The tools of quality assurance
- Standard setting
- Regulation and monitoring
- Audit
- Patient surveys and feedback

By the end of this chapter you should be able to:

- undertake evaluation of individual care interventions with the involvement of the patient
- understand the importance of evaluation and reviewing care at individual and service level
- discuss the tools and techniques that healthcare practitioners use to evaluate and review practice and services
- explain why it is important that health and social care is quality assured.

While many elements of the NMC platforms that make up the standards of proficiency for registered nurses are covered, this chapter has particular reference to (NMC, 2018b):

- Platform 4: Providing and evaluating care

- Platform 6: Improving safety and quality of care

For further detailed mapping please see *Appendix 1 – Detailed mapping to Future Nurse: standards of proficiency for registered nurses*.

7.1 Introduction

The final stage of the care process as described by Sutton (2006) is review and evaluation (*Figure 7.1*). As stated, however, the process is cyclical and continuous, as review and evaluation may lead onto further assessment, starting the process again. Evaluation is not a one-off activity but is ongoing. It is a process, where needs are continuously assessed and reassessed according to ongoing evaluation.

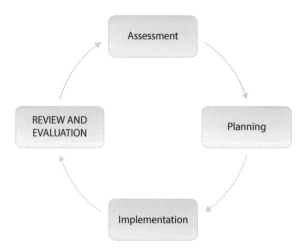

Figure 7.1 *The final phase of the ASPIRE process.*

Evaluating the effectiveness of care delivery for individuals, specific services and for society is important on a number of levels:
- Evaluation contributes to the evidence base on both an individual and population level and helps to ensure the right care interventions are used with the right individuals.
- Evaluation supports the policy drivers for the improvement of care delivery on both service and national level.
- Evaluation helps to improve care delivery in terms of quality, efficiency and effectiveness as well as safety and the prevention of health and social care disasters.

Since the inception of the NHS (and indeed before) there have been numerous documents concerned with the quality of care for patients. There is also much focus on the financial necessity to improve efficiency. This was reflected as long ago as the publication of *Clinical Governance: quality in the new NHS* (NHS Executive, 1999), and Lord Darzi's report (Department of Health, 2008a), which required professionals to improve clinical behaviours in order to improve clinical outcomes for patients. More recently, *Leading Change, Adding Value* (Department of Health, 2016) has been published as a framework to evaluate the impact of clinical outcomes based on ten commitments:

1. We will promote a culture where improving the population's health is a core component of the practice of all nursing, midwifery and care staff.
2. We will increase the visibility of nursing and midwifery leadership and input in prevention.
3. We will work with individuals, families and communities to equip them to make informed choices and manage their own health.
4. We will be centred on individuals experiencing high value care.
5. We will work in partnership with individuals, their families, carers and others important to them.
6. We will actively respond to what matters most to our staff and colleagues.
7. We will lead and drive research to evidence the impact of what we do.
8. We will have the right education, training and development to enhance our skills, knowledge and understanding.
9. We will have the right staff in the right places and at the right time.
10. We will champion the use of technology and informatics to improve practice, address unwarranted variations and enhance outcomes.

7.2 The purpose of evaluation

Evaluation simply means to assess the value of something, and this raises an interesting question – valuable in terms of what (Brophy *et al.*, 2008)? This is dependent of course on who carries out the evaluation and why it is being carried out. Within healthcare, evaluation will normally be carried out to answer the question of whether the care intervention has worked and whether the 'cost' was worth it. The difficulty is that, depending on who is concerned with the evaluation (the individual service user, the practitioner, the service provider or those who commission [pay for] the service) the question of 'is it worth it?' may have different answers. This complexity is demonstrated in *Activity 7.1*.

ACTIVITY 7.1

Herceptin is a drug now commonly prescribed as a pharmaceutical intervention for breast cancer. However, this was not always the case. Use the BBC news website to investigate the case regarding a Court of Appeal for Ms Rogers to access the drug (e.g. see http://news.bbc.co.uk/1/hi/health/4684852.stm).

Whose different perspectives in terms of evaluating the use of this drug were reported and how did they differ before the ruling to allow Ms Rogers to receive the drug?

Can you find more recent cases of this type of public debate where individual benefit and national cost implications are being played out?

In *Leading Change, Adding Value* (Department of Health, 2016) the six Cs (care, compassion, courage, communication, commitment and competence), which are a central plank of the 'Compassion in Practice' policy drawn up under the leadership of the then Chief Nursing Officer for England, are used to focus care provision across the three main principles of improving:

- health and wellbeing
- care and quality
- funding and efficiency.

The aim is to provide better outcomes, better experiences and better use of resources. In order to achieve this, care providers are asked to identify "proposed areas of unwarranted variation to be addressed" so that a standardised high-quality care provision is given.

Importantly, however, evaluations should be systematic both in terms of the process and reporting. This means that they are carried out in such a way that allows other people to follow the same process and understand how it was written up and how the results of the evaluation have been analysed (Brophy *et al.*, 2008).

7.3 Evaluating individual care

For individual service user interventions, care evaluation is about reviewing the effectiveness of care and serves two purposes:

1. It enables the healthcare practitioner to ascertain whether the desired outcomes for the client have been achieved.
2. It acts as an opportunity to review the entire process and determine whether the assessment was accurate and complete, any diagnostic element was correct, the goals of the intervention were realistic and achievable and the resulting process of implementation was successful (Hogston, 2007).

Of course the service user is not a silent partner in this process as they are not passive recipients of care. This means that healthcare practitioners must ensure that, as with every stage of ASPIRE, the voice of the service user is heard at the evaluation and review stage (see *Chapter 4*).

To review the care that is given at an individual level, it is useful to follow a series of questions about each stage of the care process. Hogston (2007) suggests a number of questions (see *Table 7.1*), which were formulated to think about nursing care.

Table 7.1 *Reviewing the Nursing Care Plan*

1. Have the short-term goals been met?
2. If so, has the diagnosis or 'problem' been resolved so that it no longer needs to be addressed?
3. If the answer is no, then why have the care goals not been met? Did they meet the MACROS criteria? (see *Section 5.2*)
4. Was the planned care intervention realistic, explicit, evidence-based, prioritised, involved and goal-centred? (REEPIG – see *Section 5.1.1*)
5. Was the method of intervention appropriate?
6. Was there effective communication within and between the care team?
7. Was the client satisfied with their care?

7.4 Quality assurance of individual care

The continuing process of review and evaluation informs the quality of care experienced by service users. Quality assurance at an individual level is determined by several factors.

7.4.1 Professional standards

The NMC is responsible for setting standards for the assessment of those wishing to enter the register and stay on it – essentially the establishment of professional competency and proficiency.

There are now seven platforms within the new standards of proficiency for registered nurses (NMC 2018b; published 2018 but introduced January 2019), which:
- represent the knowledge, skills and attributes that all registered nurses must demonstrate when caring for people of all ages and across all care settings
- reflect what the public can expect nurses to know and be able to do in order to deliver safe, compassionate and effective nursing care
- provide a benchmark for nurses from the EEA, EU and overseas wishing to join the register
- provide a benchmark for those who plan to return to practice after a period of absence.

The seven platforms (which are mapped throughout this book) are:
1. Being an accountable professional
2. Promoting health and preventing ill health
3. Assessing needs and planning care
4. Providing and evaluating care
5. Leading and managing nursing care and working in teams
6. Improving safety and quality of care
7. Coordinating care.

The NMC has also published standards for pre-registration nursing programmes. When read together with *Future Nurse: standards of proficiency for registered nurses* these give a complete picture of what nurses and midwives need to know and be able to do by the time they register, and the NMC's expectations of universities and their practice learning partners for delivering NMC-approved programmes for nurses and midwives. These focus on:

- learning culture
- educational governance and quality
- student empowerment
- educators and assessors
- curricula and assessment.

For more information see www.nmc.org.

In additional, the NMC will (from 2019) become the regulator for nursing associates (see www.nmc.org.uk/news/news-and-updates/landmark-moment-as-nmc-becomes-regulator-for-nursing-associates).

7.4.2 Implementing evidence-based practice

Clinical or non-clinical guidelines are documents that guide decisions within services based on the examination of current evidence and best practice. They summarise the consensus regarding specific interventions and also some of the practical issues involved with their implementation. They address important questions related to clinical and non-clinical practice and identify all possible options and outcomes, sometimes following decision trees or algorithms which point to decision points and possible courses of action. Guidelines are important in setting the standards for care interventions in order to improve the quality of care, and also to enable equity of provision and to ensure that the most effective and efficient treatments are used.

The National Institute for Health and Care Excellence (NICE) is an independent organisation that provides national guidance and advice to improve outcomes for people using the NHS and other public health and social care services by (see www.nice.org.uk/guidance):

- producing evidence-based guidance and advice for health, public health and social care practitioners
- developing quality standards and performance metrics for those providing and commissioning health, public health and social care services
- providing a range of information services for commissioners, practitioners and managers across the spectrum of health and social care.

NICE carries out assessments of the most appropriate practice, taking into account both patient outcomes and the financial impact using the concept of quality-adjusted life years (QALYs). Guideline Development Groups consisting of medical professionals, representatives of patient and carer groups and technical experts work together to assess the evidence base and best practice and, after a consultation period, issue guidance.

Consider Frank's diagnosis of Parkinson's disease. Visit www.nice.org.uk/guidance/conditions-and-diseases/neurological-conditions/parkinson-s-disease and consider the latest quality statements concerning the care of adults with this disease.

From the list of related NICE standards, which ones do you feel hold relevance in Frank's case?

7.4.3 Benchmarking

Benchmarking is the process of comparing the quality of what one organisation or service does against what another organisation or service does. It enables current practice to be measured against best practice and evaluated in terms of whether changes or improvements need to be made.

One example is the Essence of Care benchmarks (www.gov.uk/government/publications/essence-of-care-2010), which were first introduced in 2001 and have been frequently revised. Essence of Care 2010 is a versatile tool that can be used in a number of ways at individual and organisation level. For the evaluation and quality assurance of individual care, it can be used as a checklist of what patients, carers and staff agree is best practice in areas as diverse as:

- bladder, bowel and continence care
- care environment
- communication
- food and drink
- prevention and management of pain
- personal hygiene
- prevention and management of pressure ulcers
- promoting health and wellbeing
- record-keeping
- respect and dignity
- safety
- self-care.

There are many advantages of benchmarking and the RCN has summarised these as (Royal College of Nursing, 2017):

- providing a systematic approach to the assessment of practice
- promoting reflective practice
- providing an avenue for change in clinical practice
- ensuring pockets of innovative practice are not wasted
- reducing repetition of effort and resources
- reducing fragmentation/geographical variations in care
- providing evidence for additional resources
- facilitating multidisciplinary team building and networking
- providing a forum for open and shared learning
- being practitioner-led, and giving a sense of ownership

- accelerating quality improvement
- improving the transition of patients across complex organisational care pathways
- contributing to the NMC revalidation process (NMC, 2018a) in both reflection and CPD elements.

7.4.4 Critical incident analysis and reflective practice

Critical incident analysis involves reflecting on either good or bad practice to give insight into that practice and is not explicitly concerned with identification of ineffective or incompetent practice. This is because learning can be achieved through the identification and reflection on actions that have had positive outcomes for the care recipient. The use of critical incident analysis as a tool to improve care-giving depends on the ability of individuals to reflect upon and question practice and therefore to recognise either a dissonance between the care given and the required outcome for the care recipient, or conversely to recognise why good outcomes were achieved (Hayes and Llewellyn, 2008).

Reflective learning is a crucial part of knowledge development for professional practice, where knowledge is processed through experience. Schön's (1984) model of reflection in action has been influential in many approaches to professional development and the process by which practitioners create meaning through the observation and analysis of issues and themes that arise in practice settings.

Reflective practice is a process that must be undertaken by all Registered Nurses both personally and through the process of clinical supervision. The process of reflective practice is being used by different professional groups, with the aim of improving care through changing practice.

Reflection, however, is not new to any level of intelligent thought. Dewey defines reflective thought as that which results from an event in life that provokes or arouses a state of perplexity or uncertainty and leads the individual to search for possible explanations or solutions (Dewey, 1933). This can be applied throughout the human experience. It could be argued that it is what makes us human. Human beings plan and take actions to achieve certain outcomes, monitoring ongoing action and its consequence to make sure we achieve what we planned for!

Johns (2004) incorporated Carper's (1978) 'ways of knowing' into a model of reflection to allow the practitioner to appreciate personal, ethical and empirical influences on the experience, thereby framing learning through reflection. Johns describes (believing definition impels authority) reflection as:

> … a fusion of sensing, perceiving and intuitive thinking related to a specific experience to develop insights into self and practice. It is a vision-driven process, concerned with taking action towards knowing and realising desirable practice. (2004, pp. 2–3).

Gibbs' (1988) seminal work on the reflective cycle clearly demonstrates the cyclical and continual process of reflection (*Figure 7.2*).

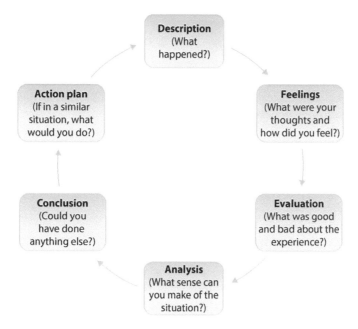

Figure 7.2 *Gibbs' reflective cycle (1988).*

The following scenario shows how Gibbs' reflective cycle might be used in practice.

REFLECTION: LIZZIE

What happened?

Lizzie was admitted to the A&E Department with a suspected stroke. I was the Nursing Assistant who was caring for her and making the initial assessment.

Feelings

I was really nervous as I had not experienced this situation before. Lizzie looked a lot like my Grandma who had just died.

Evaluation

I was pleased that I could help Lizzie and I felt close to her but it was also a bit off-putting because she reminded me of my Grandma. I felt like crying at one point and needed to leave the room.

Analysis

I know that I need to stay professional and give everyone the same kind of care and respect dignity and not make judgements about people based on appearances.

Conclusion

Instead of getting upset, I could have talked to the Nurse in Charge to explain that Lizzie looked like my Grandma and that she had just died. It might have been better to have someone more experienced with me.

Action plan

If a similar situation arises, I will definitely speak to someone to explain. I don't want other members of staff to think I am an emotional wreck and it is important that I am professional in front of relatives so that they have confidence in me.

7.5 Quality assurance of services

Much of the quality of care experienced by the individual service user is dependent on factors that are broader than the individual practitioner who is implementing the care. Quality assurance refers to planned and systematic processes that try to provide confidence in an activity or intervention or in a service or organisation's suitability for its intended purpose. Quality assurance activities aim to ensure that the services will meet requirements in a systematic, reliable way (Hayes and Llewellyn, 2008).

7.5.1 Structure, process and outcome

In a seminal work, Donabedian (1988) described a model of quality assurance for the evaluation of healthcare, which describes three aspects to specifying and measuring quality: structure, process and outcome. All three are considered equally important in measuring the quality of care provided by an organisation and they are complementary and should be used collectively to monitor quality of care.

- Structure refers to human and physical resource and can include staff and policy.
- Process refers to the methods of working, so may include the procedures for allocating resources or implementing guidelines.
- Outcomes refer to the effect of both the structure and the process, the result of a number of individual 'outputs'. The outcome relating to a clinical guideline being introduced, for example, would be improved patient care with improved clinical outcomes (Hayes and Llewellyn, 2008).

7.5.2 Quality perspectives

Hayes and Llewellyn (2008) also interpreted a model initially proposed by Huycke and All (2000) for the quality of healthcare provision (*Table 7.2*):

Table 7.2 *Model of quality perspectives (adapted from Hayes and Llewellyn, 2008)*

Perspective	Focus
Providers (healthcare organisations)	The process and outcomes of care, including having the knowledge to deliver care and achieving the required healthcare outcomes (e.g. meeting waiting list targets)
Payers (taxpayers or private insurance)	The affordability and access to care according to need
Public	Standards and regulations set by the government
Patients	Subjective view of the quality of care

7.5.3 The balanced score card approach

Another approach to quality assurance often used to evaluate whole organisations is using the balanced score card, first conceived by Kaplan and Norton in 1996. This involves grouping performance measures in general categories (perspectives) and is believed to aid organisations in the gathering and selection of the appropriate performance measures, thus contributing to quality assurance. Four general perspectives are proposed (*Figure 7.3*).

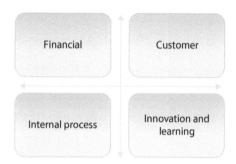

Figure 7.3 *Balanced score card approach.*

- The financial perspective within health and social care services may be one of remaining within budget and the questions that therefore need to be asked are about affordability and sustainability of interventions.
- The customer or service user perspective describes the satisfaction of the service user who receives the services.
- The internal process perspective is concerned with the processes that create and deliver the services, and considers all the activities and key processes required in order for the company or organisation to excel at providing the service effectively.
- The innovation and learning perspective focuses on the skills and capabilities that are required to deliver the required services. This is about the people who work within the services and asks whether they are trained and educated to do the job required of them, and whether the information systems are effective in enabling the organisations to keep up-to-date and informed (Kaplan and Norton, 1996).

7.5.4 Service evaluation

To assess the efficiency of a service there are different questions that can be asked:

- Is the service cost-effective?
- Are the interventions affordable and sustainable?
- Are the service users satisfied with provision (the family and friends test)?
- What do staff think about their service (staff satisfaction surveys)?

7.5.5 Regulation and monitoring

The Care Quality Commission (CQC) was established by the Health and Social Care Act 2008 (Department of Health, 2008b) and is responsible for regulating the quality of health and social care (see *Table 7.3*) and looking after the interests of individuals detained under the Mental Health Act (2007) (Department of Health, 2007; Care Quality Commission, 2008).

The CQC is responsible for registering, reviewing and inspecting services and where providers of services fail to meet the legal requirements of their registration, it has the legal powers to take action against them. The aim is therefore to enable services to improve by ensuring that essential quality and safety standards are met and where shortcomings are identified, to use enforcement powers to force organisations to improve their standards.

Table 7.3 *Care Quality Commission – 'How we do our job'*

The way we regulate care services involves:

- registering people that apply to us to provide services.
- using data, evidence and information throughout our work.
- using feedback you've given us to help us reach our judgements.
- inspections carried out by experts.
- publishing information on our judgements. In most cases we also publish a rating to help you choose care.
- taking action when we judge that services need to improve or to make sure those responsible for poor care are held accountable for it.

From www.cqc.org.uk/what-we-do/how-we-do-our-job/how-we-do-our-job

7.5.6 The audit cycle

Audit is at the heart of quality improvement, as it can be used as a tool to review and improve all services by:

- providing the mechanisms for reviewing the quality of everyday care
- building on a long history of healthcare professionals reviewing case notes and seeking ways to serve their patients better
- addressing quality issues systematically and explicitly, providing reliable information
- confirming the quality of services and highlighting the need for improvement.

(adapted from National Institute for Clinical Excellence, 2002)

Clinical audit

Clinical audit is a quality improvement process that seeks to improve patient care and outcomes through systematic review of care against explicit criteria and the implementation of change. Aspects of the structure, processes and outcomes of care are selected and systematically evaluated against explicit criteria. Where indicated, changes are implemented at an individual, team or service level and further monitoring is used to confirm improvement in healthcare delivery.

Clinical audit can be described as a cycle or a spiral. Within the cycle there are stages that follow a systematic process of establishing best practice, measuring care against criteria, taking action to improve care, and monitoring to sustain improvement. The spiral suggests that as the process continues, each cycle aspires to a higher level of quality (National Institute for Clinical Excellence, 2002).

Figure 7.4 shows an example of the audit cycle (www.qualityinoptometry.co.uk).

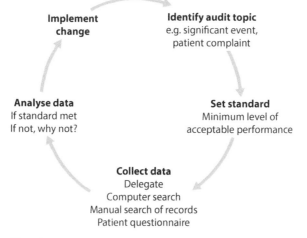

Figure 7.4 *The audit cycle.*

ACTIVITY 7.3

You work as a Nursing Associate in a GP practice and the manager has asked you to be involved in an audit about patient satisfaction. She would like to gather some data around how patients rate your service when you have provided some aspect of care for them. The topic area is about communication and you need to think about the best ways to get some honest and useful feedback about your service provision, so that you can continually improve care to patients.

What ideas can you think about?

Are there any constraints to getting valuable information?

Use SMART (see *Chapter 5*) to design a short and easy-to-complete survey.

Try to think about how you would get Frank and Lizzie to provide information.

Implementing change

The Plan, Do, Study, Act (PDSA) model is a basic service improvement model and is a common tool for implementing change (*Figure 7.5*). The four stages of the PDSA cycle are:

- **Plan** – the change to be tested or implemented
- **Do** – carry out the test or change
- **Study** – data before and after the change and reflect on what was learned
- **Act** – plan the next change cycle or full implementation.

(NHS Institute for Innovation and Improvement, 2011)

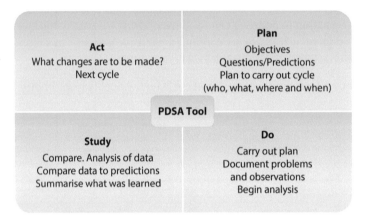

Figure 7.5 *Diagrammatic representation of the PDSA tool.*

ACTIVITY 7.4: FRANK AND LIZZIE

Think back to Frank and Lizzie.

As you know, Lizzie is feeling more and more socially isolated as her and Frank's physical and mental health deteriorates. Plan a single intervention that may help them to feel less isolated and follow the PDSA cycle to evaluate your approach.

The NHS has also designed its Change Model to assist in improving services (see www.england.nhs.uk/sustainableimprovement/change-model/). The three key ideas on which the NHS Change Model is based are worth considering to ensure that any change is effective and sustainable as an improvement. They are:

1. Intrinsic and extrinsic motivators for change
2. Anatomy and physiology of change
3. Balancing commitment and compliance.

ACTIVITY 7.5

Visit the NHS Change Model website (www.england.nhs.uk/sustainableimprovement/change-model/) for resources, webinars and forums – which are constantly being updated.

The Change Model frequently asked questions page provides a standard slide set, and a downloadable picture of the NHS Change Model.

You can also contribute to discussions on Twitter using #nhschange.

7.5.7 Serious incident analysis and service user safety

Recognition that incidents or adverse care events cannot be eliminated from complex modern healthcare has been an important step in recent years in learning from such events to improve future service user safety. Indeed one of the things that might result in an audit being undertaken is an Untoward Incident. In 2000 the Department of Health published its paper 'Organisation with a Memory' (Department of Health, 2000) to formalise the process of collecting and analysing accurate data on adverse healthcare events, leading to the creation in 2001 of the National Patient Safety Agency (NPSA). The NPSA has the responsibility of improving the safety and quality of patient care through reporting, analysing and disseminating the lessons of adverse events and 'near misses' involving NHS patients.

The format for doing so is based on the process of:
- gathering information on the root cause of the incident (i.e. identify the factors that led to the hazard occurring)
- learning from it (i.e. study and consult widely)
- acting to prevent it happening again (identify interventions which may prevent reoccurrence) and so preventing or reducing risk.

ACTIVITY 7.6

All clinical areas receive relevant national patient safety incident reports (NaPSIRs). Research the latest one to be circulated to your clinical area. What happened and what changes are expected as a result of the alert?

In addition to the NPSA, the Medicines and Healthcare products Regulatory Agency (MHRA) was created and is the government agency responsible for ensuring that medicines and medical devices work and are acceptably safe.

ACTIVITY 7.7

The MHRA monitors safety and quality standards of medicines and medical devices in several ways, for example regular inspections to ensure good and safe practice in:
- manufacturers and suppliers of medicines and medical devices
- medicines distribution and storage
- clinical trials
- clinical inspecting systems for devices
- laboratories testing medicines
- auditing notified bodies
- blood establishments.

Visit the MHRA website (www.gov.uk/government/organisations/medicines-and-healthcare-products-regulatory-agency) and investigate in what other ways it contributes to the safety of service users.

Family members often witness the care given to patients and may judge the care to be good or below the standard expected. This can inform the quality assessment of care or it may become even more significant. The science behind ergonomics or human factors is an emerging discipline for healthcare and lessons learned in other industries (especially aviation) have started to become embedded. Martin Bromiley's wife Elaine was admitted to hospital for routine surgery and died as a result of 'human factors'. Martin was an aircraft pilot and was familiar with the science of human factors and wanted answers to questions about the death of his wife. He has become a pioneer for human factors in healthcare and founded the charity Clinical Human Factors Group (CHFG), which champions patient safety.

ACTIVITY 7.8

Search online for Martin Bromiley and look at the CHFG website (www.chfg.org/) to find more information on human factors in healthcare. Identify one human factor that you have seen contributing to poor care. What action could be taken to prevent that happening again?

7.5.8 Serious child safeguarding practice reviews

Serious child safeguarding cases are those in which abuse or neglect of a child is known or suspected and the child has died or been seriously harmed. The nature of Child Safeguarding Practice reviews is set out in Chapter 4 of the document *Working Together to Safeguard Children* (HM Government, 2018).

Serious harm includes (but is not limited to) serious and/or long-term impairment of a child's mental health or intellectual, emotional, social or behavioural development. It should also cover impairment of physical health. This is not an exhaustive list. When making decisions, judgement should be exercised in cases where impairment is likely to be long-term, even if this is not immediately certain. Even if a child recovers, including from a one-off incident, serious harm may still have occurred.

The purpose of serious child safeguarding reviews is to:
- establish whether there are lessons to be learned from the case about the way in which local professionals and agencies work together to safeguard and promote the welfare of children
- identify clearly what those lessons are, how they will be acted on, and what is expected to change as a result; and consequentially
- improve inter-agency working and better safeguard and promote the welfare of children.

Serious safeguarding practice reviews may also be undertaken where an adult has died and there is suspicion or evidence of neglect or abuse, as in the case of Steven Hoskin, who was a 39-year-old man with learning disabilities. He was subjected to systematic abuse by carers, who hauled him round his bedsit with a dog collar, burned him with cigarettes and eventually made him cling to a viaduct, where he fell to his death after being kicked in the face and having his hands stamped on. Although Steven Hoskin was known to social services, insufficient action was taken to safeguard him from this abuse.

ACTIVITY 7.9

Read the summary of the serious case review into a child in Camden by scanning the QR code on the right, or visiting bit.ly/Activity7-9.

What lessons can be learned to improve future practice?

There are Safeguarding Adults Boards that work strategically to improve the provision of care for vulnerable adults (see www.tsab.org.uk/ as an example of a regional adult safeguarding board).

7.5.9 Service user and carer surveys and feedback

Service user and carer satisfaction is one factor taken into consideration for judging quality of care, and service user and carer surveys and feedback are being increasingly used in healthcare services. Organisations can gather user feedback in a variety of ways including surveys (Friends and Family), audits, comments and complaints, focus groups and interviews. Health and social care organisations are mandated to undertake user surveys and actively seek feedback. By constantly and systematically surveying care, a detailed picture of the experience of service users is drawn. National surveys are valuable as they allow local organisations to compare the performance of similar organisations across the country. It also means it is possible to identify the things that really matter to service users. The Picker Institute, for example, which is commissioned to survey the NHS, has found that the things that are most important to service users are (Picker Institute, 2009):

- fast and reliable health advice
- effective treatments delivered by trusted professionals
- participation in decisions and respect for preferences
- clear, comprehensive information and support for self-care
- attention to physical and environmental needs
- emotional support, empathy and respect
- involvement of and support for family and carers
- continuity of care and smooth transitions.

In addition to service user and carer surveys, Patient Reported Outcome Measures (PROMs) are a method of collecting information on the quality of clinical care as reported by service users themselves. Service users answer the same set of questions on their quality of life before and after an operation and the comparable data is then used to calculate a numerical value for the improvement to their health. The focus for this approach started with all licensed providers of hip replacements and reports can be seen at the NHS website (www.digital.nhs.uk/data-and-information/data-tools-and-services/data-services/patient-reported-outcome-measures-proms).

CHAPTER SUMMARY

This chapter focused on the evaluation and review stage of ASPIRE. It is essential that healthcare practitioners understand the importance of evaluating health and social care at individual service user level, organisational level and national level. There are many contemporary policy drivers and a plethora of tools and techniques that can be used in order to ensure that care is effectively quality assured and evaluated.

Reflection

Identify at least three things that you have learned from this chapter.

1. ....
....
2. ....
....
3. ....
....

How do you plan to use this knowledge within clinical practice?

1. ....
....
2. ....
....
3. ....
....

How will you evaluate the effectiveness of your plan?

1. ....
....
2. ....
....
3. ....
....

What further knowledge and evidence do you need?

1. ....
....
2. ....
....
3. ....
....

FURTHER READING

Aveyard, H. and Sharp, P. (2017) *A Beginner's Guide to Evidence Based Practice in Health and Social Care*, 3rd edition. London: Open University Press.

This is the book for anyone who has ever wondered what evidence-based practice is, how to relate it to practice or use it in academic work. It provides a step-by-step guide to what we mean by evidence-based practice and how to apply this concept to your practice and learning.

Fully updated in this edition, this book uses simple and easy-to-understand language to help those new to the topic.

Brophy, S., Snooks, H. and Griffiths, L. (2008) *Small-Scale Evaluation in Health: a practical guide*. London: Sage.

Setting out the basics of designing, conducting and analysing an evaluation study in healthcare, the authors take a practical approach, assuming no previous knowledge or experience of evaluation. All the basics are covered, including: how to plan an evaluation; research governance and ethics; understanding data; interpreting findings; writing a report. Case studies are included throughout to demonstrate evaluation in action, and self-learning courses give the reader an opportunity to develop their skills further in the methods and analysis involved in evaluation.

Conklin, T. (2012) *Pre-Accident Investigations: an introduction to organizational safety*. Boca Raton, FL: CRC Press.

This is a new way to explore why untoward events happen and embraces concepts from human factors science.

Health Education England, short film 'Raising Concerns':

www.youtube.com/watch?v=zjau1Ey0di8

Heaslip, V. and Lindsay, B. (2019) *Research and Evidence-Based Practice*. Banbury: Lantern Publishing.

This accessible and easy-to-read text enables students to understand what research is and how it can provide evidence for practice. It uses clear explanations, key case studies, questions and activities to explore the principles of research needed for students to develop their own evidence-based practice. It covers areas such as why research is carried out and why it matters, and gives thorough guidance on how to search and review the literature in order to evaluate the quality of research. It explores how research projects are designed and participants recruited, how data is collected and analysed, and how research findings are communicated. It also covers important areas related to the cost and funding of research, ethics, and how to review evidence and use it to improve the quality of care. For the student, it has a practical and applied approach that enables the development of ways to both demonstrate the understanding of research and evidence, and to develop and promote best practice in health and social care.

Teeswide Safeguarding Adults Board website:

www.tsab.org.uk/

The NHS Change Model:

www.england.nhs.uk/sustainableimprovement/change-model/

Chapter 8
Conclusion and future challenges

LEARNING OUTCOMES

Throughout the book, we have introduced the ASPIRE framework as a systematic approach to shape nursing care and provided examples to help you to apply this framework in practice and develop your skills. However, as discussed in *Chapter 1*, this is very much influenced by the context of health and social care policy. This chapter will build on the discussion in *Chapter 1* and explore some of the challenges that impact on nursing care in the 21st century. For this reason, this chapter is slightly more theoretical to help you to develop critical knowledge and understanding of the policy context that impacts on the ASPIRE process and nursing care.

This chapter covers the following key issues:

- Contemporary social processes that affect demand and need for care.
- Current policy imperatives in healthcare.
- Definitions of power and the context within which power operates and influences care provision.
- Factors that impact on collaborative and partnership working.
- Digital transformations and the impact on care.
- Where power can lead to abuse.

By the end of this chapter you should be able to:

- understand the factors that influence the nature of healthcare provision
- explain how issues of power might impact on the ASPIRE process
- examine issues that impact on user involvement in decision-making processes in healthcare
- reflect on the impact of the digital world on health and nursing care
- reflect on the nature of the power that is held by healthcare professionals and its potential for doing harm.

While many elements of the NMC platforms that make up the standards of proficiency for registered nurses are covered, this chapter has particular reference to (NMC, 2018b):

- Platform 1: Being an accountable professional

- Platform 6: Improving safety and quality of care

- Platform 7: Coordinating care

For further detailed mapping please see *Appendix 1* – Detailed mapping to *Future Nurse: standards of proficiency for registered nurses*.

8.1 Introduction

Health and social care services are witnessing a period of radical transformation, with a move away from a professionally led model of service delivery to person-centred care, based on individual assessment of needs and the provision of services to promote independent living wherever possible. The emphasis in both adult and children's health and social care provision is on the empowerment and rights of individuals, and there is an increased emphasis on ensuring that vulnerable children and adults are safeguarded from abuse and harm. This all takes place within a wider context and is impacted by processes of globalisation, changing demographics and the information age, as discussed in *Chapter 1*. For example, the issues around modern slavery and 'mate and hate' crime are relatively new concepts that need consideration by healthcare professionals.

8.2 Globalisation

The process of globalisation is a complex range of activities, not just a single activity, which provide a social and political context for everyday lives and institutional processes. There are contested definitions of globalisation (Dominelli, 2007), but a common definition identifies a process of increasing global interconnectedness, whereby goods and services, capital flow and workers increasingly move around the world, encouraged by trade and revolutions in communications and technology (Martell, 2010). Globalisation therefore refers to processes of economic, political and ideological interconnectedness, involving global networks of markets, communications and increased movement of people between countries and continents. One reason for the growth of globalisation in the last two decades has been the growth of information and communication technologies, which have facilitated this interconnectedness and the ease of communication between distant localities with a resulting high level of access to information that we may not have historically had access to.

ACTIVITY 8.1: FRANK AND LIZZIE

Think of Frank and Lizzie, when they were young adults. There was no internet, or television, and limited news through the radio and print media. How would their knowledge of global events be different from today? If they wanted to know more about symptoms or a disease they were concerned about, how would they get information about it?

Globalisation has also led to new areas of social oppression and exclusion generated through the displacement of people through immigration and emigration and increased vulnerability through lifestyle and consumer practices (Harrison and Melville, 2010). The global context of social disadvantage can be seen in the high levels of psychosis in migrant groups (Morgan and Hutchinson, 2010). This has been related to high levels of stress and uncertainty within the social, political and economic context of poverty and migration, with migrant workers (including those working in healthcare) encountering new forms of risk (Christensen and Manthorpe, 2016).

The subtlety of modern slavery means it is easily missed. For example, if you use a nail bar to have your nails manicured, would you recognise signs of slavery? (There is guidance at www.gov.uk/government/publications/modern-slavery-awareness-booklet).

The demographic factors discussed in *Chapter 1* have led to increasing demand for healthcare at a time when expenditure on public services is under scrutiny. Between 2003/04 and 2015/16 the number of hospital admissions in the UK increased by 3.6% per year. The demand for healthcare has also led to more acutely ill admissions with shorter in-patient stays and quicker discharges. Funding for healthcare is slowing down and not keeping pace with increasing demand and needs, leading to an imbalance between supply and demand (King's Fund, 2017). Sepsis is more common in older adults than any other age and older adults with 'frailty' require much more intense care than ever before. So as the demographics show, as the number of older people increases, the demand for resources will escalate at a time when fewer young people will be available to care for them.

Resource issues are a constant challenge in a health and social care environment where demographic changes and changing expectations are placing increasing demands on service providers. This is particularly pertinent in times of economic recession, with increased scrutiny of public expenditure in relation to statutory services, and raises issues about the operation of the mixed economy of welfare and the effective and efficient use of both individual and organisational budgets.

A second challenge for health and social care professionals stems from policies that aim to increase independent living and social inclusion. Since the 1990 National Health Service and Community Care Act, there has been an emphasis on maximising independent living in adult social care, and this has been further strengthened through the personalisation agenda and self-directed support.

There are also challenges in terms of workforce development and the training, education, monitoring and regulation of service providers (including people paid as personal assistants within the personalisation and independent living agenda).

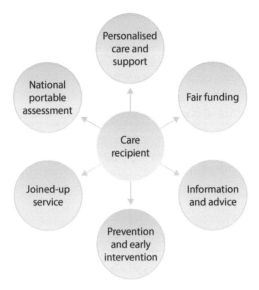

Figure 8.1 *Key policy imperatives from* Shaping the Future of Care Together *(Department of Health, 2009).*

To address these challenges, successive governments have undertaken a programme of modernisation of public services. Underpinning this modernisation agenda is the notion of consumerism and the active participation of consumers in the delivery and monitoring of services, with a shift in the power dynamic from service provider to service consumer. This has resulted in the Health and Social Care Act (Department of Health, 2012a), which was built on in the 2014 policy document *Five Year Forward View* (Department of Health, 2014b) and again in the NHS Long Term Plan launched in January 2019.

Assessment and good planning of care in conjunction with the service users and their carers is crucial to improving the quality of care for all and requires a fundamental shift in attitudes to reflect this new focus on self-assessment and addressing needs as the recipients of services identify them. Whilst these transformations offer positive ways of working and valuing people, they also pose a number of challenges for professionals working within health and social care, as well as for service users and their carers.

8.3 **Technological change**

Globally, there has been a technological revolution throughout the latter half of the 20th century and continuing into the 21st century (Macionis & Plummer, 2012), which has led to fundamental changes in societal organisation in every aspect of life, including health and social care provision. People have access to electronic devices in their daily communications through the use of computers, mobile devices and smartphones, which is mediated through the infrastructures of broadband, wireless communication and libraries of electronic information. According to the Office for National Statistics (2019), virtually all adults aged 16 to 44 years in the UK were recent internet users (99%) in 2019, compared with 47% of adults aged 75 years and over, with the 16–24 year age group spending most time online in recreational and leisure activities, including social networking.

This technological revolution can be seen in healthcare provision. These changes have had a significant impact on the context and delivery of healthcare. For example, in *Chapter 6* we looked at the concept of stress and how this can be managed. It might be worth considering how stress can be managed using technology. There are numerous apps designed to help relieve stress such as the 'Headspace' app, which has a free 10-day beginner's course and uses mindfulness techniques with the aim of helping to reduce stress.

Robotics is another area where considerable developments are taking place. For example, it is already possible to buy robotic floor cleaners and these could help disabled people to maintain a clean and safe environment. Robotics and artificial intelligence have far-reaching implications for the transformation of healthcare from prevention through to intervention (*Figure 8.2*).

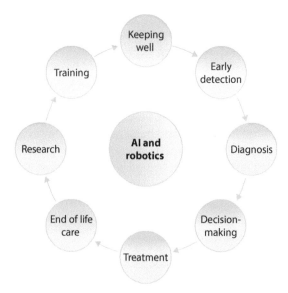

Figure 8.2 *Potential impact of AI and robotics on healthcare (adapted from www.pwc.com/gx/en/industries/healthcare/publications/ai-robotics-new-health/transforming-healthcare.html).*

We have recently seen a proliferation of wearable technologies to monitor blood pressure, exercise and diet, which demonstrates this trend towards the use of AI and robotics in healthcare. We can also see this in the case study of Stephen Hawking, the British theoretical physicist who died in March 2018 at the age of 76. He was diagnosed with a rare form of motor neurone disease at 21 and given two years to live. The disease led to progressive paralysis and loss of speech. However, he was able to continue to communicate through a speech-generating device that was operated through his cheek muscle.

The information age has also led to increased access to a wide range of health advice and information. The proliferation of health information on the internet has led to a dramatic increase in people using this as their first source of health information (Tan and Goonawardene, 2017). The relevance of consumer health informatics is likely to increase. For example, health and social care providers are exploring how 'consumers' engage in service provision. In recent times, the emergence of ambulatory centres (walk-in centres) was an attempt to provide care facilities outside hospital A&E Departments to alleviate some of the pressures on them. It can be argued that the ambulatory centres in fact increased demand rather than reducing pressures. Many centres are now closing and GP surgeries are trying to use facilities more effectively. Service providers are evaluating how people access and engage with the services in light of widely available digital technology.

Other countries are also addressing this issue and it is worth looking at the Singapore Smart Nation template for a glimpse into what is possible in the UK. Technological developments therefore offer new ways of working and can be positive in terms of new networking opportunities and developments in independent living, but offer challenges in relation to resources and partnership working.

8.3.1 Social inclusion and empowerment through independent living – the role of assistive technologies

Assistive technologies can provide effective support to empower individuals for more independent living. Assistive technologies provide challenges in terms of a shift in ways of working, but at the same time provide enormous opportunities for maximising people's independence and helping them to stay in their own homes or preferred place of care. The document *Front Line Care: the future of nursing and midwifery in England* (Prime Minister's Commission, 2010) gave 20 recommendations including using technology in healthcare. Some of the recommendations are still relevant and the examples used in the report are pertinent. For example, on page 31, it gives an outline for care of a patient, Mary, who has a long-term condition and how her care might be managed in 2020.

Information technology can enhance people's sense of citizenship and social participation through opening up opportunities for interaction, through email and other forms of online communication. It can also empower people to manage their own finances, shopping and other personal affairs rather than being dependent on others.

AGE UK HELPS OLDER PEOPLE SAVE ONLINE
(ITea and Biscuits, evaluated 2012)

Saving money and finding good deals are a priority for increasing numbers of older people as the financial downturn deepens. In response to this demand, Age UK's **'ITea and Biscuits'** programme included guidance and training about online shopping during internet training and advice sessions. Read a blog about it here: www.ageukblog. org.uk/tag/itea-and-biscuits/

The programme helped older people to use online shopping, which can save money, and price comparison sites, which allow people to research and make buying decisions within the comfort of their home. Online shopping also saves pensioners from having to carry goods home and already four in ten retired people are regular e-shoppers. Many older people ask specifically to learn about eBay and how it can help them generate cash and find bargains. Internet usage has overtaken gardening and DIY as a hobby for pensioners, who spend an average of six hours a week online.

Silversurfers (www.silversurfers.com/) is a group that was established to demonstrate the benefits of technology for supported living, increasing independence and providing greater choice and control and social capital for older people. There is an active online forum for Silversurfers, who exchange information and suggestions using technology. Information on its website is accessible and easy to navigate and covers a wide range of interest areas.

While there are positive aspects to enhanced technology use, it should be remembered that digital exclusion can be exacerbated through poor access to technology, whether this is in terms of access to software and hardware, user patterns, user skills or the availability of social support systems (Rourke and Coleman, 2011). Effective use of new technologies is also contingent upon having a health and social care workforce that is adequately educated and trained to work in collaboration with service users and carers and signpost appropriate services to meet their needs. All of these challenges are relevant to the ASPIRE process, as the transformations in ways of working with both adults and children require a fundamental shift in professional attitudes and the balance of power between professionals and service users and carers.

8.4 Power

The concept of power is central to the challenges of assessing, planning, implementing and evaluating health and social care in the 21st century and underpins many of the issues outlined above. So what do we mean when we talk about power and how does this relate to health and social care practice? Power is a term that is frequently used in all walks of life, but as a theoretical concept it is difficult to define. There is no single definition of power and it will mean different things in different social contexts, but it is useful to look at a number of different elements that are related to the concept of power.

Power is all around us and is a pervasive element of social relations, operating between individuals as well as through social organisations, political groups and formal institutions (Gubbay, 1997). When exploring power, therefore, it is important to understand the social context that it operates in as well as the outcome of the actions.

ACTIVITY 8.2

Make a list of the ways in which power has been used within your life. (When you've finished reading this chapter, go back to this list and think about any additions that you would make.)

Think about the role of a health or social care practitioner when assessing the care needs of an individual.

Who holds the power?

What factors contribute to a power imbalance in health and social care?

Power is an important concept in health and social care, as individuals and groups that engage with services may be disadvantaged through disempowerment in a number of ways. The concept of oppression is related to power, and serves to limit an individual's participation in the decision-making process. Oppression can be defined as a "system of interrelated barriers and forces that reduce, immobilise and mould people who belong to a certain group in ways that effect their subordination to another group" (Kendall, 1992).

The following groups, who are significant users of health and social care services, have been particularly powerless and oppressed in society (Thompson, 2007):
- People with mental health problems
- People with learning disabilities
- People with physical disabilities
- People with long-term conditions
- Children (especially looked-after children)
- Older people
- People who are homeless
- Ex-offenders.

The concept of psychological or personal power can be used to further explore disempowerment and oppression. This affects the individual's ability to achieve their goals and to address their own needs or make their own decisions and is related to the skills, attributes, roles and attitudes that the individual has (Thompson, 2007).

When thinking about power and people with mental health problems or people who have learning difficulties, it is worth considering how vulnerable people can be radicalised into terror activities. The UK PREVENT strategy is a way to highlight to health and social care staff the indicators that vulnerable people are being radicalised. The training course 'HealthWrap' gives important information and advice for care staff about what to do if they suspect a service user is a victim of radicalisation (see www.elearning.prevent.homeoffice.gov.uk/).

8.4.1 Skills

The exercising of power is affected by the individual's skills, such as communication or assertiveness. As discussed in *Chapter 2*, communication is central to the ASPIRE process and the skill of good communication can empower people within the care-giving process. This involves thinking about how the communication will be received by the patient (and their carer) and adapting accordingly.

ACTIVITY 8.3

Think about the following words/phrases that health and social care practitioners might use:

"Are you managing to feed yourself OK?"

"Do you drink enough?"

"How is your pain today?"

- Is the interpretation clear?
- What alternative interpretations might people put on these phrases?
- Can you see that the questions have an underlying assumption that the service user is eating/drinking and has pain?
- How easy would it be for the service user to answer with a one-word response (yes/ yes/OK)?
- These questions won't give any indication about how much the person is eating/ drinking or suffering.
- How would the person be able to say whether they were eating enough, etc., and how would you know their assessment is evidence-based/accurate?
- How could the questions be posed differently?

Thus communication and the way people use language is an important aspect of power and disempowerment, and impacts on the ways that people use health and social care services and the extent to which they feel empowered to make their own decisions and engage in the processes of care. Overlooking or misinterpreting communication with children can lead to them either being excluded from the decision-making process, or erroneous decisions being made (Jones, 2003), and effective communication with children is emphasised as a priority in professional education programmes for nurses (Sully and Dallas, 2010). There is a growing body of research exploring ways of reaching people whose voices have not traditionally been heard (see *Chapter 2*).

People may also be disempowered as they lose skills. Returning to the case study of Frank and Lizzie, we can see that Frank is struggling with some of the functional skills of daily living, such as eating, speaking and mobilising (see *Chapter 1*). The skill of the nurse is in finding adaptations and tools that can empower Frank to manage these functions independently. For example, the nurse could discuss an appropriate diet for Frank and Lizzie that minimises the need for him to cut up hard foods such as meats and discuss the use of different eating implements that might make it easier for him to eat independently. It is important to use the skills of other members of the multidisciplinary team, such as dietitians, for specific advice for individuals.

8.4.2 Attributes

The personal characteristics of an individual may affect their ability to exert power, because of the ideological constructions of society. This means that through discourses and social reproduction (the ways that people talk about and accept situations as normal and are happy for that approach to continue), society constructs ideas about the relative value of different attributes, leading to the construction of dominant groups. For example, it is argued that Western societies are somatic societies, with a focus on the body and constructions of the normal/abnormal body and the relative worth and value of the individual (Llewellyn *et al.*, 2015). Historically people with disabilities or impairments were segregated into institutions as they were seen as abnormal; this segregation contributed to a fear of the unknown and people with disabilities came to be seen as inferior and people to be feared, leading to stereotyping and marginalisation.

Similarly, in a society that places value on youth, older people are stereotyped on the basis of their physical appearance, and stereotypical assumptions are made about physical and mental deterioration, contributing to financial and social marginalisation. The body therefore is an important site of power and control and those who are devalued on the basis of physical attributes are marginalised and disempowered in social relations. This can be extended to the value placed on people in terms of perceived mental ability and stereotypical assumptions about an individual's behaviour and participation.

A number of health conditions are stigmatised in society, which involves a process of social labelling, leading to devaluing and negative attitudes. Vulnerable people who are supported to live independently can be easily targeted by criminals and 'mate and hate crime' is a relatively new concept to describe how vulnerable people can be befriended by criminals and bullied into actions they are not comfortable about (for more information, see www.mencap.org.uk/advice-and-support/bullying/mate-and-hate-crime).

"When I applied for a job as a cleaner at a care home the manager called me and wanted to know more about my disability, which I'd declared. She pressed me so I said "I'll be absolutely open with you. I've got a schizoaffective disorder and I hear three voices of people I knew." There was complete silence on the phone. She didn't say a word. So I said "Hello, are you still there?" All she said was, "I'll be in touch." Anyway, a few days later, lo and behold, I received a rejection letter. To me her silence spoke volumes and I felt very discriminated against."

Extract from Department of Health (2006e) *Action on Stigma* (available by scanning the QR code on the right)

What stereotypes are apparent here?

What are the implications of this negative social labelling in terms of power?

The marginalisation and stigmatisation of people is related to disempowerment within the care processes, and health and social care professionals need to take this into account when engaging service users in the assessment and planning of care needs. Health and social care professionals also need to be aware of their own values and the influence that wider social issues may have in terms of stereotypical assumptions about a service user's abilities and skills. A model of reflective practice and self-reflexivity is important in helping practitioners to critically reflect on their own value base and explore ways that this might impact on the ASPIRE process (see *Chapter 7*).

8.4.3 Roles

People have different roles in society and these roles are ranked hierarchically based on the social construction of value. This is partly related to attributes as discussed above, but also relates to dominant sets of ideas, where dominant groups are able to use power to perpetuate this hierarchical division to further their own advantage. Society is divided on class, gender and ethnic lines as well as constructions of age, sexuality and ability (Llewellyn *et al.*, 2015).

It should also be remembered that there may be crossover between these categories. For example, an older person may also be homeless, or suffer from mental health problems. In addition, their degree of power may be further influenced by the social variables of class, gender, ethnicity and sexuality.

Consider the scenario where a nurse and a doctor disagree about the best way to treat a patient.

What sort of factors in terms of their roles might influence the power dynamic here?

8.4.4 Attitudes

Peoples' own attitudes can affect their ability to exert power and control over their own lives. Issues such as confidence, self-esteem and willingness to take risks are all important indicators of a person's attitude and ability to take control. Self-esteem can be influenced by a number of factors, including how we perceive ourselves and how others see and value us, and it is closely related to our levels of confidence.

LIZZIE

Take, for example, the case study of Lizzie. Since breaking her ankle and suffering with a detached retina, she has increasingly lost confidence and is reluctant to take risks for fear of inflicting more damage. This has led to poor self-esteem and limits the activities that Lizzie is engaged in.

Inner resources and life cycle experiences are important contributors to people's attitudes and sense of power, but so too are the environments and structures within which those experiences are shaped. The social construction of dominant ideas may have a powerful impact on people as they come to internalise those dominant value systems and may therefore see themselves as not having the ability to do something.

ACTIVITY 8.6

Frank and Lizzie's estranged daughter visits. While they are delighted that there may be a reunion in sight, Lizzie becomes more and more concerned that the daughter is trying to persuade Frank and Lizzie to move into long-term care, saying that her sister is not coping and needs a break.

What factors of power may be at play here?

What motivations can you identify here?

Power can therefore be seen as the power to do something based on personal and psychological processes, but it is also related to wider social structures and institutional practices and power over other people. The development of a professional-led model of care (see *Chapter 1*) focused power in the hands of welfare professionals, who had the power to define needs, assess people's level of needs and plan and deliver interventions based on eligibility criteria and availability of services. Although the model of healthcare delivery is changing to one that is more person-centred and user-led, funding arrangements and eligibility criteria still reflect dominant power relations, which limit the publicly-funded support that can be provided.

Power is therefore a concept that applies to the influence that people are able to exert over others. This is sometimes referred to as ideological power (the extent to which individuals can influence dominant sets of ideas in society) or structural power (the extent to which individuals are empowered within the structures and institutions of society to exert control over others) (Gramsci, 1971). A good example of this is the power that the medical profession has had in the assessment of needs and the biomedical approach to assessing people for services, as discussed in *Chapter 1*.

8.4.5 Abuse

All types of power, including that which healthcare professionals hold, can also lead into more specific examples of abuse, where a person in a position of power uses that position to cause harm (physical or otherwise) to the individual in their care or influence. Abuse is a very serious crime and a complete betrayal of professional standards. For more information on what constitutes abuse please see *Appendix 4* and *Table 8.1*, which examines why people abuse adults.

Table 8.1 *Why do people abuse adults?*

Five personality types of perpetrators:
1. **Domineering or bullying** perpetrators feel justified in abusing others. These people usually know where and when they can get away with abusive behaviour.
2. **Narcissistic** (means inflated sense of own importance, and lack of empathy for others) people are motivated by anticipated personal gain and meeting their own needs, and do this by using other people and their assets. This could include inheriting an elderly person's home, gaining access to benefits or stealing other valuables.
3. **Impaired** perpetrators are well-intentioned care-givers who have problems that mean they are unable to adequately care for dependent adults. This includes advanced age and frailty, physical and mental illness and developmental disabilities.
4. **Overwhelmed** perpetrators are well-intentioned care-givers in personality, intelligence, skills and motivation. However, when pressure mounts for them to provide more than they are capable of, they lash out verbally or physically and/or the quality of their care may degrade to the point of neglect. Risk factors include stress and depression and social isolation.
5. **Sadistic** perpetrators derive feelings of power and importance by humiliating, terrifying and harming others. They take pleasure in their victim's fear and don't feel guilt, shame or remorse (sadistic means getting pleasure from inflicting pain, suffering or humiliation).

Adapted from Dr Holly Ramsey-Klawsnik (2000), from www.tsab.org.uk/general-public/

8.4.6 Organisational hierarchy and power

Weber (1976) used the term rational-legal authority to describe the power that individuals have within organisations. He was interested in how complex organisations are structured to achieve their goals, and used the term bureaucracy to describe an organisation that is structured according to hierarchical division of offices, with a top-down chain of command and a set of rules to govern behaviour and practices within the organisation. Those who hold higher positions in the hierarchy are seen to have legitimate power and authority by virtue of their position.

This theory remains relevant for understanding the way that complex organisations such as the NHS are organised and can be seen in new managerialist systems of organisation that have been implemented as part of the modernisation agenda in health and social care (Glasby, 2017). Whilst bureaucracies may be seen as the epitome of rational legal authority within institutions, they have also been criticised for the overemphasis on rules and procedures. For example, there have been criticisms that health and social care services have become too focused on achieving the targets and performance criteria to measure the performance of the organisation (Pollock and Talbot-Smith, 2006) at the expense of assessing the needs of individuals and providing a person-centred service. Parry-Jones and Soulsby (2001) have argued that needs-led assessment is difficult to pursue in practice, where practitioners continue to be gatekeepers to scarce resources. Hence, there may be more emphasis on the needs of the organisation than on the needs of the individual service user, with eligibility criteria being used as a way of rationing resources.

ACTIVITY 8.7

Breaching waiting lists

There are a number of ways that priority for admission to hospital or eligibility for care services can be managed:

1. First-come, first-served basis
2. Assessment of clinical priority
3. Ability to pay

Which system fits best with Weber's concept of rational-legal authority?

What are the implications of these different systems for efficient management of welfare services?

Read the article by Goddard and Tavakoli (2008) for a more detailed discussion of management of waiting lists.

Abstract

A queuing model for public health service waiting lists is developed, and the implications for patient welfare of different systems for managing the waiting list are analysed. If patients are admitted to hospital on a first-come, first-served basis, a welfare gain is achieved by moving from a system of implicit to one of explicit rationing of access to the waiting list. If individual waiting times and hospital admissions are dependent on clinical priority, a further welfare gain is achievable without the use of explicit rationing, by reallocating the total waiting time from the more towards the less seriously ill. On efficiency and welfare criteria, a maximum waiting time guarantee does not appear to be a desirable development.

Power therefore operates at an organisational and structural level and this can impact on the care process. Power also operates at the level of individuals and is an important aspect of social relationships. As discussed in *Chapter 4*, differentials in power at this individual level can impact on the assessment process.

8.4.7 Ways in which individuals may exercise power

1. Persuasion – an individual may be persuaded to do something by another person because of their superior status. Thus within a hierarchical system of organisation, people who are seen to have authority by virtue of their superior position in the hierarchy can persuade subordinates of appropriate courses of action.

ACTIVITY 8.8: FRANK AND LIZZIE

Frank and Lizzie's estranged daughter has not been to visit for several months. She turns up at their house one day and tells them that her son is starting an apprenticeship in the building industry and needs to buy some new tools. She asks Frank what has happened to his tools since he can no longer use them for DIY.

Consider the elements of persuasion in this case.

2. People may be induced to behave in a certain way. For example, a service user may be induced to comply with a professional assessment of needs or plan of intervention for fear of being labelled unpopular (Stockwell, 1972) or not receiving any services.
3. Anticipated reaction – people may do or not do something in anticipation of a reaction from another person. People may therefore behave in a way that they would not otherwise have done in order to get the reaction that they want or feel is expected of them. For example, a person may appear grateful for a prescription, when they have no intention of taking the pills, as they feel that this is what the doctor or nurse expects of them.
4. Disciplinary power – the normal workings of society constantly reaffirm and reproduce the existing power structures through registration, inspection, certification, surveillance and individuation. Thus nurses have power by virtue of their registration as professionals and the certification of their knowledge base.
5. Habituation – this is where the person is so used to complying that it is done automatically. An example of this is where a person becomes institutionalised with loss of liberty and freedom and an emphasis on organisational priorities rather than individual needs.

ACTIVITY 8.9

Tony works as a healthcare assistant in a care home. He has only been there for a couple of months, and does not agree with the manager's practice of insisting that all the residents have a rest period straight after lunch. However, he goes along with the practice, as he feels uncomfortable about challenging the manager, particularly as all other staff seem happy to comply.

What elements of habituation AND persuasion are apparent here?

Power can lead to institutional practices that disempower residents/patients. King and Raynes (1968) identify four features of an institution:
- depersonalisation
- social distance between staff and residents
- block activities, where activities are rigidly organised at a group level, providing little opportunity for individuals to state their preferences
- a lack of variety in daily routine.

Hospitals, care homes and group homes may all be examples of institutions, but service users may also become institutionalised within their own homes where organisational processes limit their freedoms.

ACTIVITY 8.10

Read the following extract:

"Once in the lounge patients had to be removed again at regular intervals to be reordered or taken to the toilet. Then they went to lunch, back to bed for two hours, up again for late tea, to the toilet, into dinner, to the toilet, to the lounge, to the toilet and finally to bed. During the night, auxiliaries undertook two-hourly rounds in which each patient was checked and their body ordered as necessary." (Lee-Treweek, 1997, p. 54)

In what ways are the patients institutionalised?

In what ways do staff exercise power?

How are the patients disempowered?

What could be done differently so that residents could exert more power?

Power then can affect the interpersonal relationship and the way that the ASPIRE process operates. However, power can also be used to provide benefits for service users. We can use the term 'power with' to explore the concept of power within society. 'Power with' refers to the power derived from working together in partnership or collaboratively with other individuals (see *Chapter 5*). This power can be seen in the development of user and carer groups who have become involved in decision-making at all levels of health and social care delivery. As discussed throughout this book, user involvement and person-centred care remain a continuing policy priority in health and social care, but variations in service user involvement across service user groups as well as between different organisations and service providers remain. Achieving user involvement in health and social care decision-making and in both shaping their own health and social care needs and the wider context of provision continues to present a challenge for health and social care professionals. The challenge is to build on models of good practice, so that there is true service user and carer involvement in decision-making, assessment and service provision, with true partnerships in care, rather than tokenistic involvement.

The disability movement has been influential in shaping services and demonstrates the power of pressure groups. See, for example, the work of Disability Rights UK, who campaign for equal participation for all (www.disabilityrightsuk.org/about-us).

However, there are also groups of service users whose voices are rarely heard and who continue to be marginalised, with minimal or absent involvement in the decision-making process.

8.4.8 Barriers to service user participation

- Power – unequal power relationships or perceptions about levels of power can limit service user involvement.
- Differing priorities – although there is a move towards personalisation and person-centred care, it has been argued that in reality, health and social care professionals may continue to assess people for services and act as gatekeepers

to public services. This means that rather than addressing service user needs and implementing a plan of care to address these needs, people are fitted into existing services, on the basis of a one-size-fits-all approach, which is counter to person-centred care (Parry-Jones and Soulsby, 2001).

- Relationships between individuals and organisations where equity was an issue have limited the involvement of some service users in health and social care.

For example, in the report *Breaking the Circles of Fear*, which remains as relevant and important today as when it was published, the Sainsbury Centre for Mental Health (2002) found that many black people experienced poor-quality services in mental health care, as stereotypical views, racism and a lack of cultural awareness contributed to poor assessment of needs, and subsequent treatments dominated by interventions, including a heavy reliance on medication and restriction. This poor experience of care led to people being reluctant to seek treatment, which increased the likelihood of personal crisis and reinforced the stereotypical views of staff, where service users were perceived as potentially dangerous. The recommendations of the report are summarised as follows:

- Ensure that black service users are treated with respect and that their voices are heard.
- Deliver early intervention and early access to services to prevent escalation of crises.
- Ensure that services are accessible, welcoming, relevant and well integrated with the community.
- Increase understanding and effective communication on both sides, including creating a culture which allows people to discuss race and mental health issues.
- Deliver greater support and funding to services led by the black community.

These recommendations have been operationalised through various initiatives and policy directives, achieving change through working with service users and gateway organisations. Good service user involvement encompasses engaging service users at every level of service provision, including education and training.

SHAPING OUR LIVES

Shaping Our Lives is a user network that promotes collaborative working between service users and health and social care agencies. Its website (www.shapingourlives.org.uk) states its aims:

- "to support the development of local user involvement that aims to deliver better outcomes for service users
- to give a shared voice to user controlled organisations
- to facilitate service user involvement at a national level
- to work across all user groups in an equal and accessible manner
- to improve the quality of support people receive
- to enable groups to link to other user-controlled groups
- to develop links with world-wide international user-controlled organisations."

Alongside the challenge to engage service users within a needs-led system of care delivery, there are also challenges to engage carers in the stages of the decision-making process. Walker and Dewar (2001) summarise satisfactory carer involvement in decision-making as follows:

- Feeling that information has been shared with them.
- Feeling included within the decision-making process (see earlier reference to Arnstein's 'ladder of citizenship participation' in *Section 3.4.3*).
- Feeling that there is someone who can be contacted if the need arises. This is part of the preventative and early intervention priority outlined in *Shaping the Future of Care Together* (Department of Health, 2009) and is an important aspect of empowerment.
- Feeling that the service is responsive to their needs. This can be related to the needs-led assessment and is an important aspect of assessment frameworks such as the Single Assessment Process. This can also be seen in policy developments, as discussed in *Chapter 2*.

CHAPTER SUMMARY

This chapter has examined the need and delivery of care within contemporary social processes by examining current policy imperatives in healthcare. By defining power and examining the context within which power operates and influences care provision, we have examined factors that impact on collaborative and partnership working, including the transformation seen within an age of digital technological advancement. We have also explored how power can lead to discrimination and abuse and so proposed that a radical transformation of health and social care services requires a cultural change in attitudes from service users and carers and professionals, with challenges to unequal power relationships as well as expectations about the way that services are developed and delivered. We have also placed an emphasis on the question of how safeguarding vulnerable people has to be balanced against empowering people to make their own decisions and to take positive risks.

FURTHER READING

Department of Health (2016) *Leading Change, Adding Value*. Available from: www.england.nhs.uk/wp-content/uploads/2016/05/nursing-framework.pdf (accessed 9 May 2019).

This publication is introduced by the Chief Nursing Officer, Jane Cummings, as a framework that every nursing, midwifery and care professional, in all settings, can use to ensure that we achieve the best quality of experience for our patients and people, the best health and wellbeing outcomes for our populations, and use finite resources wisely to get best value for every pound spent.

MENCAP – stories written by individuals with learning disabilities (www. mencap.org.uk/stories).

Mencap's stories are told by service users about their experiences of care. They include both positive and challenging scenarios where things did not go so well and are a good source for all of us to reflect on how care experiences affect the people in our care.

Glasby, J. (2017) *Understanding Health and Social Care*, 3rd edition. Bristol: Policy Press.

This is a very accessible book that explores a number of the key issues that have been discussed in this chapter. There are chapters on partnership working in health and social care, independent living and the social model of disability and user involvement in health and social care. Concepts are illustrated through clear explanations supported by tables and diagrams to highlight key points, and at the end of each chapter there are some suggestions for further reading to develop understanding of the different concepts.

Appendix 1
Detailed mapping to *Future Nurse: standards of proficiency for registered nurses*

The seven platforms for the NMC's standards of proficiency have been mapped to the chapters in this book. The main headings for the chapters lend themselves to some of the platforms but some of the details may be found in other chapters.

Please note that the platforms should be read in conjunction with the Annexe A and Annexe B components of the standards (www.nmc.org.uk/standards/standards-for-nurses/standards-of-proficiency-for-registered-nurses) but it is not the remit of this text to explore nursing procedures in depth.

Platform and components	Most relevant chapters
Platform 1 – Being an accountable professional	Introduction
1.1 understand and act in accordance with the Code (2018): *Professional standards of practice and behaviour for nurses, midwives and nursing associates*, and fulfil all registration requirements	3
1.2 understand and apply relevant legal, regulatory and governance requirements, policies, and ethical frameworks, including any mandatory reporting duties, to all areas of practice, differentiating where appropriate between the devolved legislatures of the United Kingdom	5
1.3 understand and apply the principles of courage, transparency and the professional duty of candour, recognising and reporting any situations, behaviours or errors that could result in poor care outcomes	5
1.4 demonstrate an understanding of, and the ability to challenge, discriminatory behaviour	7
1.5 understand the demands of professional practice and demonstrate how to recognise signs of vulnerability in themselves or their colleagues and the action required to minimise risks to health	8

(continued)

Platform and components	Most relevant chapters
1.6 understand the professional responsibility to adopt a healthy lifestyle to maintain the level of personal fitness and wellbeing required to meet people's needs for mental and physical care	1
1.7 demonstrate an understanding of research methods, ethics and governance in order to critically analyse, safely use, share and apply research findings to promote and inform best nursing practice	3
1.8 demonstrate the knowledge, skills and ability to think critically when applying evidence and drawing on experience to make evidence informed decisions in all situations	6
1.9 understand the need to base all decisions regarding care and interventions on people's needs and preferences, recognising and addressing any personal and external factors that may unduly influence their decisions	3
1.10 demonstrate resilience and emotional intelligence and be capable of explaining the rationale that influences their judgments and decisions in routine, complex and challenging situations	3
1.11 communicate effectively using a range of skills and strategies with colleagues and people at all stages of life and with a range of mental, physical, cognitive and behavioural health challenges	2
1.12 demonstrate the skills and abilities required to support people at all stages of life who are emotionally or physically vulnerable	2
1.13 demonstrate the skills and abilities required to develop, manage and maintain appropriate relationships with people, their families, carers and colleagues	2
1.14 provide and promote non-discriminatory, person-centred and sensitive care at all times, reflecting on people's values and beliefs, diverse backgrounds, cultural characteristics, language requirements, needs and preferences, taking account of any need for adjustments	2
1.15 demonstrate the numeracy, literacy, digital and technological skills required to meet the needs of people in their care to ensure safe and effective nursing practice	3
1.16 demonstrate the ability to keep complete, clear, accurate and timely records	7
1.17 take responsibility for continuous self-reflection, seeking and responding to support and feedback to develop their professional knowledge and skills	7

(continued)

Platform and components	Most relevant chapters
1.18 demonstrate the knowledge and confidence to contribute effectively and proactively in an interdisciplinary team	2
1.19 act as an ambassador, upholding the reputation of their profession and promoting public confidence in nursing, health and care services, and	8
1.20 safely demonstrate evidence-based practice in all skills and procedures stated in Annexes A and B.	6
Platform 2 – Promoting health and preventing ill health	1
2.1 understand and apply the aims and principles of health promotion, protection and improvement and the prevention of ill health when engaging with people	1
2.2 demonstrate knowledge of epidemiology, demography, genomics and the wider determinants of health, illness and wellbeing and apply this to an understanding of global patterns of health and wellbeing outcomes	1
2.3 understand the factors that may lead to inequalities in health outcomes	1
2.4 identify and use all appropriate opportunities, making reasonable adjustments when required, to discuss the impact of smoking, substance and alcohol use, sexual behaviours, diet and exercise on mental, physical and behavioural health and wellbeing, in the context of people's individual circumstances	1
2.5 promote and improve mental, physical, behavioural and other health related outcomes by understanding and explaining the principles, practice and evidence-base for health screening programmes	1
2.6 understand the importance of early years and childhood experiences and the possible impact on life choices, mental, physical and behavioural health and wellbeing	1
2.7 understand and explain the contribution of social influences, health literacy, individual circumstances, behaviours and lifestyle choices to mental, physical and behavioural health outcomes	1
2.8 explain and demonstrate the use of up to date approaches to behaviour change to enable people to use their strengths and expertise and make informed choices when managing their own health and making lifestyle adjustments	1

(continued)

Platform and components	Most relevant chapters
2.9 use appropriate communication skills and strength based approaches to support and enable people to make informed choices about their care to manage health challenges in order to have satisfying and fulfilling lives within the limitations caused by reduced capability, ill health and disability	2
2.10 provide information in accessible ways to help people understand and make decisions about their health, life choices, illness and care	3
2.11 promote health and prevent ill health by understanding and explaining to people the principles of pathogenesis, immunology and the evidence-base for immunisation, vaccination and herd immunity, and	1
2.12 protect health through understanding and applying the principles of infection prevention and control, including communicable disease surveillance and antimicrobial stewardship and resistance.	1
Platform 3 – Assessing needs and planning care	4
3.1 demonstrate and apply knowledge of human development from conception to death when undertaking full and accurate person-centred nursing assessments and developing appropriate care plans	5
3.2 demonstrate and apply knowledge of body systems and homeostasis, human anatomy and physiology, biology, genomics, pharmacology and social and behavioural sciences when undertaking full and accurate person-centred nursing assessments and developing appropriate care plans	4
3.3 demonstrate and apply knowledge of all commonly encountered mental, physical, behavioural and cognitive health conditions, medication usage and treatments when undertaking full and accurate assessments of nursing care needs and when developing, prioritising and reviewing person-centred care plans	4
3.4 understand and apply a person-centred approach to nursing care, demonstrating shared assessment, planning, decision making and goal setting when working with people, their families, communities and populations of all ages	3
3.5 demonstrate the ability to accurately process all information gathered during the assessment process to identify needs for individualised nursing care and develop person-centred evidence-based plans for nursing interventions with agreed goals	3
3.6 effectively assess a person's capacity to make decisions about their own care and to give or withhold consent	3

(continued)

Platform and components	Most relevant chapters
3.7 understand and apply the principles and processes for making reasonable adjustments	4
3.8 understand and apply the relevant laws about mental capacity for the country in which you are practising when making decisions in relation to people who do not have capacity	3
3.9 recognise and assess people at risk of harm and the situations that may put them at risk, ensuring prompt action is taken to safeguard those who are vulnerable	8
3.10 demonstrate the skills and abilities required to recognise and assess people who show signs of self-harm and/or suicidal ideation	8
3.11 undertake routine investigations, interpreting and sharing findings as appropriate	3
3.12 interpret results from routine investigations, taking prompt action when required by implementing appropriate interventions, requesting additional investigations or escalating to others	3
3.13 demonstrate an understanding of co-morbidities and the demands of meeting people's complex nursing and social care needs when prioritising care plans	5
3.14 identify and assess the needs of people and families for care at the end of life, including requirements for palliative care and decision making related to their treatment and care preferences	4
3.15 demonstrate the ability to work in partnership with people, families and carers to continuously monitor, evaluate and reassess the effectiveness of all agreed nursing care plans and care, sharing decision making and readjusting agreed goals, documenting progress and decisions made, and	5
3.16 demonstrate knowledge of when and how to refer people safely to other professionals or services for clinical intervention or support.	5
Platform 4 – Providing and evaluating care	6
4.1 demonstrate and apply an understanding of what is important to people and how to use this knowledge to ensure their needs for safety, dignity, privacy, comfort and sleep can be met, acting as a role model for others in providing evidence based person-centred care	6
4.2 work in partnership with people to encourage shared decision making in order to support individuals, their families and carers to manage their own care when appropriate	3

(continued)

Platform and components	Most relevant chapters
4.3 demonstrate the knowledge, communication and relationship management skills required to provide people, families and carers with accurate information that meets their needs before, during and after a range of interventions	2
4.4 demonstrate the knowledge and skills required to support people with commonly encountered mental health, behavioural, cognitive and learning challenges, and act as a role model for others in providing high quality nursing interventions to meet people's needs	5
4.5 demonstrate the knowledge and skills required to support people with commonly encountered physical health conditions, their medication usage and treatments, and act as a role model for others in providing high quality nursing interventions when meeting people's needs	7
4.6 demonstrate the knowledge, skills and ability to act as a role model for others in providing evidence-based nursing care to meet people's needs related to nutrition, hydration and bladder and bowel health	4
4.7 demonstrate the knowledge, skills and ability to act as a role model for others in providing evidence-based, person-centred nursing care to meet people's needs related to mobility, hygiene, oral care, wound care and skin integrity	4
4.8 demonstrate the knowledge and skills required to identify and initiate appropriate interventions to support people with commonly encountered symptoms including anxiety, confusion, discomfort and pain	5
4.9 demonstrate the knowledge and skills required to prioritise what is important to people and their families when providing evidence-based person-centred nursing care at end of life including the care of people who are dying, families, the deceased and the bereaved	7
4.10 demonstrate the knowledge and ability to respond proactively and promptly to signs of deterioration or distress in mental, physical, cognitive and behavioural health and use this knowledge to make sound clinical decisions	4
4.11 demonstrate the knowledge and skills required to initiate and evaluate appropriate interventions to support people who show signs of self-harm and/or suicidal ideation	7
4.12 demonstrate the ability to manage commonly encountered devices and confidently carry out related nursing procedures to meet people's needs for evidence-based, person-centred care	6

(continued)

Platform and components	Most relevant chapters
4.13 demonstrate the knowledge, skills and confidence to provide first aid procedures and basic life support	3
4.14 understand the principles of safe and effective administration and optimisation of medicines in accordance with local and national policies and demonstrate proficiency and accuracy when calculating dosages of prescribed medicines	3
4.15 demonstrate knowledge of pharmacology and the ability to recognise the effects of medicines, allergies, drug sensitivities, side effects, contraindications, incompatibilities, adverse reactions, prescribing errors and the impact of polypharmacy and over the counter medication usage	4
4.16 demonstrate knowledge of how prescriptions can be generated, the role of generic, unlicensed, and off-label prescribing and an understanding of the potential risks associated with these approaches to prescribing	Not explicitly addressed
4.17 apply knowledge of pharmacology to the care of people, demonstrating the ability to progress to a prescribing qualification following registration, and	Not explicitly addressed
4.18 demonstrate the ability to co-ordinate and undertake the processes and procedures involved in routine planning and management of safe discharge home or transfer of people between care settings.	5
Platform 5 – Leading and managing nursing care and working in teams	3
5.1 understand the principles of effective leadership, management, group and organisational dynamics and culture and apply these to team working and decision-making	3
5.2 understand and apply the principles of human factors, environmental factors and strength-based approaches when working in teams	2
5.3 understand the principles and application of processes for performance management and how these apply to the nursing team	5
5.4 demonstrate an understanding of the roles, responsibilities and scope of practice of all members of the nursing and interdisciplinary team and how to make best use of the contributions of others involved in providing care	5

(continued)

Platform and components	Most relevant chapters
5.5 safely and effectively lead and manage the nursing care of a group of people, demonstrating appropriate prioritisation, delegation and assignment of care responsibilities to others involved in providing care	3
5.6 exhibit leadership potential by demonstrating an ability to guide, support and motivate individuals and interact confidently with other members of the care team	5
5.7 demonstrate the ability to monitor and evaluate the quality of care delivered by others in the team and lay carers	5
5.8 support and supervise students in the delivery of nursing care, promoting reflection and providing constructive feedback, and evaluating and documenting their performance	Not explicitly addressed
5.9 demonstrate the ability to challenge and provide constructive feedback about care delivered by others in the team, and support them to identify and agree individual learning needs	5
5.10 contribute to supervision and team reflection activities to promote improvements in practice and services	5
5.11 effectively and responsibly use a range of digital technologies to access, input, share and apply information and data within teams and between agencies, and	8
5.12 understand the mechanisms that can be used to influence organisational change and public policy, demonstrating the development of political awareness and skills.	8
Platform 6 – Improving safety and quality of care	7
6.1 understand and apply the principles of health and safety legislation and regulations and maintain safe work and care environments	8
6.2 understand the relationship between safe staffing levels, appropriate skills mix, safety and quality of care, recognising risks to public protection and quality of care, escalating concerns appropriately	8
6.3 comply with local and national frameworks, legislation and regulations for assessing, managing and reporting risks, ensuring the appropriate action is taken	7
6.4 demonstrate an understanding of the principles of improvement methodologies, participate in all stages of audit activity and identify appropriate quality improvement strategies	7

(continued)

Platform and components	Most relevant chapters
6.5 demonstrate the ability to accurately undertake risk assessments in a range of care settings, using a range of contemporary assessment and improvement tools	7
6.6 identify the need to make improvements and proactively respond to potential hazards that may affect the safety of people	7
6.7 understand how the quality and effectiveness of nursing care can be evaluated in practice, and demonstrate how to use service delivery evaluation and audit findings to bring about continuous improvement	7
6.8 demonstrate an understanding of how to identify, report and critically reflect on near misses, critical incidents, major incidents and serious adverse events in order to learn from them and influence their future practice	7
6.9 work with people, their families, carers and colleagues to develop effective improvement strategies for quality and safety, sharing feedback and learning from positive outcomes and experiences, mistakes and adverse outcomes and experiences	7
6.10 apply an understanding of the differences between risk aversion and risk management and how to avoid compromising quality of care and health outcomes	7
6.11 acknowledge the need to accept and manage uncertainty, and demonstrate an understanding of strategies that develop resilience in self and others, and	7
6.12 understand the role of registered nurses and other health and care professionals at different levels of experience and seniority when managing and prioritising actions and care in the event of a major incident.	7
Platform 7 – Coordinating care	**5**
7.1 understand and apply the principles of partnership, collaboration and interagency working across all relevant sectors	5
7.2 understand health legislation and current health and social care policies, and the mechanisms involved in influencing policy development and change, differentiating where appropriate between the devolved legislatures of the United Kingdom	8
7.3 understand the principles of health economics and their relevance to resource allocation in health and social care organisations and other agencies	7

(continued)

Platform and components	Most relevant chapters
7.4 identify the implications of current health policy and future policy changes for nursing and other professions and understand the impact of policy changes on the delivery and coordination of care	7
7.5 understand and recognise the need to respond to the challenges of providing safe, effective and person-centred nursing care for people who have co-morbidities and complex care needs	8
7.6 demonstrate an understanding of the complexities of providing mental, cognitive, behavioural and physical care services across a wide range of integrated care settings	7
7.7 understand how to monitor and evaluate the quality of people's experience of complex care	7
7.8 understand the principles and processes involved in supporting people and families with a range of care needs to maintain optimal independence and avoid unnecessary interventions and disruptions to their lives	8
7.9 facilitate equitable access to healthcare for people who are vulnerable or have a disability, demonstrate the ability to advocate on their behalf when required, and make necessary reasonable adjustments to the assessment, planning and delivery of their care	8
7.10 understand the principles and processes involved in planning and facilitating the safe discharge and transition of people between caseloads, settings and services	7
7.11 demonstrate the ability to identify and manage risks and take proactive measures to improve the quality of care and services when needed	7
7.12 demonstrate an understanding of the processes involved in developing a basic business case for additional care funding by applying knowledge of finance, resources and safe staffing levels, and	7
7.13 demonstrate an understanding of the importance of exercising political awareness throughout their career, to maximise the influence and effect of registered nursing on quality of care, patient safety and cost effectiveness.	8

Appendix 2
The use of collaboration – an example

You are in the basement of a building and there are three light switches.

You are told that there are three bulbs, one on each floor (ground floor, first floor and second floor).

You need to find out which light switch connects to which bulb. The bulbs are not visible to you until you go onto each floor.

You can only go upstairs once.

How will you determine which switch is responsible for which bulb?

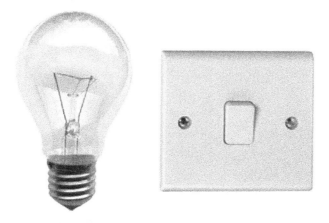

The answer – turn on two of the three light switches and wait five minutes, then turn one off.

Go up to the ground floor. If the light there is on, that means it's connected to the switch that you left on in the basement. If it's off and cold, it's connected to the switch that was never turned on in the basement. If it's off and warm, it is connected to the switch that was on for five minutes and then switched off. Check the first and second floor bulbs in the same way until you know which switch operates which bulb.

Appendix 3
The Single Assessment Process

Single Assessment Process Overview Assessment					
Contact and assessment details					
Family name:	Smith		First name:	Frank	
Preferred name:	Frank		Date of birth:	8.10.1934	
NHS number	345291	Social care number	22/39874	Telephone number	01972 382974
Assessor	Nicola Jones		Role	Staff Nurse	
Team/Ward	16		Telephone number	Ext 2396	
Assessment method	Telephone ☐ Face to face ☐ x		Assessment location	On the ward	
Assessment date	12-12-20		Other present	Wife Lizzie	
Brief description of person's presenting problems, difficulties or concerns					

Frank was diagnosed with Parkinson's disease and early-stage dementia three years ago.

Diagnosed with skin cancer and had a tumour removed from face one year ago. Cancer has spread and he had to have a large tumour resected from neck, resulting in some nerve damage (partial paralysis of one side of his face). Difficulty eating, drinking and talking. He had courses of radiotherapy and chemotherapy and has had further tumours removed from his scalp. Pre-operatively, he had to have a number of teeth removed and he now has dentures (mouth sore). He has been deaf for some years and wears hearing aids in both ears. The paralysis of his mouth has led to problems with dribbling. He has lost a lot of weight and looks malnourished and frail. Has memory loss, tremors and mobility problems.

Frank and his wife still attend Salvation Army services when they can get someone to pick them up, but no longer feel able to play the active role that has always been a fundamental part of their lives.

Formal care/support currently received (frequency, nature of support, adequacy, etc.)		
None		
Nursing/community matron		*nil*
Occupational therapy		*nil*
Physiotherapy		*nil*
Dietetic		*nil*
Podiatry		*nil*
Medical care (GP, etc.)		*Care from GP*
Social care		*nil*
Lifeline/telecare		*nil*
Psychiatry/CPN/CMHN		*Cognitive impairment, early-onset dementia, no input from Mental Health for Older People*
Speech and language		*Very hard of hearing. He was fitted with new hearing aids by the audiologist at the local hospital.*
Home care (Council funded)		*None*
Day care		*None*
Other (specify)		*Have filled out the Lasting Power of Attorney paperwork to authorise their son and eldest daughter to make decisions on their behalf.*

| Name: | *Frank Smith* | | | Date of birth: | *08.10.34* |

Assessment key: Y = Problem/need or yes; **N** = No need/problem or **No?** = Possible problem; **N/A** = Not applicable; **N/K** = Not known; **U =** Unassessed

Sensory and communication

Eyesight	*y*			
Hearing	*y*			
Speech/expression	*y*			
Understanding	*y*			
Other problem *(specify)*	*dyslexia*			

Medical history (recent admission in the last 28 days; recent procedures or falls in past year)

Recent admission?	*y*	
Recent procedure?	*y*	
Recent falls?	*y*	
Long-term condition?	*y*	
Main diagnosis?	*Parkinson's disease*	
Additional diagnosis?	*skin cancer*	
Other problem *(specify)*	*cognitive impairment*	

Physical wellbeing

Physical wellbeing	*y*	
Weight loss/gain	*y*	
Appetite/diet	*y*	
Allergies	*n*	
Pain	*y*	
Skin (including pressure areas)	*y*	
Breathing	*n*	
Seizures/epilepsy	*n*	
General foot health	*n*	
Swallowing	*mouth ulcers*	
Oral health status/dental	*ulceration and sinister 'lumps' in mouth*	

Name	Frank Smith	Date of birth	8.10.34	Completed by	N Jones
Bowels	n				
Continence (urine)	n				
Continence (faeces)	n				
Blood pressure	n				
Temperature, pulse, respiration	n				
Other problem (specify)	n				

Health Screening

Alcohol intake (units per week)	n	Smokes (number per day)	0
Routine screening	n	*Frank is not eating sufficient calories and protein.*	
Fluid intake	?		
Diet/intake	n		
Vaccinations	n		
Exercise	n		
Sexual health	n		

Physical health needs identified? *If yes, consider further tests and/or referral e.g. for check-up.*

Assessment Key: **Y** = Problematical or yes. **N** = No needs or problem. **No?** = Possible problem. **N/A** = not applicable. **N/K** = not known

Psychological wellbeing

Reaction to bereavement/ loss	?	*Frank has some cognitive impairment and may not easily verbalise pain. Frank has become more forgetful and his GP has asked him to attend the memory clinic for assessment.*
Depressed mood	y	
Irritability	y	
Lowering of energy, drive and interest	y	
Sleep	y	

Memory	y								
Orientation	y								
Anxiety/phobias	y								
Indicators of severe mental illness	y								
Risk behaviours	n								
Substance misuse	n								
Self-neglect	y								

Mental health needs identified? *If yes, consider further tests and/or referral e.g. for check-up.*

Medication

Current medication (including non-prescribed – specify)	None taken		Takes medication (see below)

Co-beneldopa 600mg daily

Galantamine 12mg twice a day

Paracetamol 1gm every 6 hours

Ordering/collecting medications	y	Has dosette box that pharmacist prepares for him. Evidence that he does not always remember to take his medication.
Taking medication as prescribed	?	
Managing label/containers	?	
Swallowing medicines	y	
Uses medication aids?	y	
Pharmacist support	y	
Medication reviewed in past year?	y	*If no, arrange GP review, if not known check with GP*

Needs in relation to medication identified? If yes, make arrangements for review or appropriate referral		

Assessment Key: **Y** = Problematical or yes. **N** = No needs or problem. **No?** = Possible problem. **N/A** = not applicable. **N/K** = not known		

Interpersonal relationships (recent means the past year)		
Level of social contact	y	*Committed Salvationist who ran a homeless shelter for some time and Frank finished his career as a prison chaplain working with young offenders. He formally retired from this role when he was 80.*
Level of carer contact	n	
Family/carer relationships	y	*Has four children, one son and three daughters, all of whom now have families of their own. Their son is their eldest, lives some distance away, he is in regular contact and visits them when he can. Eldest daughter lives about five miles away and they see her regularly. She helps with shopping and cleaning. The youngest child lives some distance away, in regular contact and visits once a month.*
Other relationships	y	
Caring for others	y	
Child protection issues	n	

Name:	*Frank Smith*	Date of birth:	*8.10.34*	Completed by:	*N Jones*

Adult protection issues	*y*	Some evidence of unintentional neglect and medicine mismanagement.
Recent victim of crime?	*n*	
Other problem *(specify)*	*n*	

Social circumstances

Finances

Income and benefits	*y*
Problems receiving benefits	*n*
Finance management	*n*

Activities and employment

Problems to employment	*n*	*Frank left school at the age of 14 with no qualifications. Profoundly dyslexic, always been extremely practical, e.g. built summerhouse as well as fitting the kitchen and bathroom. He has had a number of jobs, including farm worker, milkman and taxi driver.*
Access to employment	*n*	
Access to education	*n*	
Access to training	*n*	
Access to other activities	*y*	
Access to services/amenities	*n*	

Housing situation

Location of housing	*outskirts of town*	*Lives with wife in a two- bedroomed bungalow in which they have lived very independently.*
Type of housing	*2 bed bungalow*	
Security/type of tenure	*owner*	
Access to home	*okay*	
Access within home	*okay*	

Home environment

Amenities	*n*	Bath and shower – all on 1 floor. Shower over the bath. This may make it difficult for Frank to get into as his mobility decreases.
Heating	*y*	
Existing adaptation	*n*	
Working smoke alarm	*y*	
General repair/condition	*good*	

| Name | *Frank Smith* | Date of birth | *8.10.34* | Completed by | *N Jones* |

Social needs identified? If yes, consider appropriate further assessments and/or referral

| **Activities of Daily Living** | **Overall ADL Score** | | **5** |

0 = Fully independent. No assistance required from another person. May use equipment, adaptations, Telecare etc. No need for support.	3 = Limited independence. Always requires assistance, supervision or prompting to undertake activity. (Other person must be present.)
1 = Largely independent. Occasional reminder or prompting required and/ or difficulties in undertaking requiring occasional help (include phone calls). Person not usually required to be present.	4 = High dependency. Does not or cannot undertake activity. Requires activity to be undertaken by one other person.
2 = Partial independence. Often requires assistance, supervision or prompting (other person must be present). Can sometimes undertake independently.	5 = High dependency. Does not or cannot undertake activity. Requires two or more people to undertake activity.

Self-care

Eating/drinking	2
Washing	2
Bathing	2
Toileting – day time	1
Dressing/undressing	2
Grooming	2

Everyday needs

Cooking/food preparation	2
Domestic tasks	2
Shopping	2

Mobility (inside the home)

Moving	2						
Going up/down stairs	3						
Getting on/off chair	2						
Getting into/out of bed	2						
Turning in bed	1						
Lying to sitting	1						
Toileting (night time)	2						
Minimum level of assistance required	None			1 person	x	2 people	

Name	*Frank Smith*	Date of birth	*8.10.34*	Completed by:	*N Jones*

Does the person use aids, equipment or adaptations to support independence?							*no*

Has a decline in skills been observed?	*yes*	By person	*wife*	By carer		By assessment/ review	

Frank is becoming increasingly frail physically and mentally, looking towards end-of-life care.

Can the person respond to emergencies?	No	x	Yes			To a limited extent	

Needs in ADLs identified? If yes, consider OT assessment/referral and/ or continuing care pre-screening

Assessment key: **Y** = *Problem/need or yes.* **N** = *No need/problem.* **N?** = *Possible problem.* **N/A** = *Not applicable.* **N/K** = *Not known*

Prior assessment and needs informing this assessment

Type	Date	Assessor	Role	Results and comments
Blood pressure				*BP 110/63* *P 72 bpm*
Diabetes screening and assessment				*R 14/min* *T 36.4 C* *BM = 4.5 mmols/l*
Lay assessment				*MMT – not completed* *Frailty - yes*

| Name: | *Frank Smith* | Date of birth: | *8.10.34* | Completed by: | *Social worker* |

Other contributions to this assessment *(via direct contribution or liaison. Who and what?)*

Skin cancer has likely spread, suspected secondaries.

| **Risk arising** *(assessor's view of risk – note differences with person/carer.)* | *2* |

Risk score

- 0 = No apparent risk. No history/warning signs indicative of risk.

- 1 = Some apparent risk (no previous history). No history indicative of risk but current factors/warning signs indicate possibility of risk.

- 2 = Some apparent risk (with previous history). History indicative of risk and current factors/warning signs suggest presence of risk.

Risk of falling	2
Risk re. physical condition	2
Domestic risk *(e.g. fire)*	1
Risk loss of autonomy	1
Risk to daily activities/routine	1
Risk to relationships	0
Risk of social isolation	0
Risk of abuse/neglect by others	0
Risk of severe self-neglect	0
Risk related to wandering	0
Risk of suicide	0
Risk of deliberate self-harm	0
Risk of others from person	0
Risk medication management	1
Moving/manual handling risk	1
Risk of pressure sores	1
Risk of carer support	1

Strengths and protective factors/Potential for self-care *(e.g. personal qualities, social support)*

Wife is finding it increasingly difficult to cope.

Name:	*Frank Smith*	Date of birth:	*8.10.34*	Completed by:	Social worker

Summary of person's views/priorities

Frank has limited understanding about his future care needs; he thinks 'all will be okay'. Wife is worried and can see Frank deteriorating and thinks that 'the cancer has come back'.

Summary of carer's views/priorities

Lizzie would like more support and does not want to be so reliant on her family. She finds it difficult to cope with her inability to cope as well as she once did.

Assessor's summary *(including overall impact of needs on person's independence, quality of life)*

Probably looking at terminal care, Frank scores high on the frailty assessment score. No active investigation into cancer spread but terminal care needs seem evident.

Key needs identified	FACS Level (ASSD Only)
Medicine assessment	x
Refer to PD Specialist Nurse	x
Check memory clinic review date	x
Carer support needed	Assessment booked
Social worker referral to see if help with finances can be arranged	No

FACS eligibility *(Adult social care)*

None		Low		Moderate	x	Substantial		Critical	

| Name | Frank Smith | Date of birth | 8/10/34 | Completed by | N Jones |

Further actions

Have direct payments been discussed?	No	x	Yes but not required			Yes and required	
Continuing care indicated?	No				Yes	x	

No further action		Refer for carers' assessment to see if further support needed.
Information and advice		
Ongoing monitoring	x	Refer for OT assessment re adaptations in bathroom.
Referral(s) (indicate reasons)	x	
Liaise with (indicate reasons)	x	
Assessments (indicate reasons)	x	
Care plan/carer support plan	x	
Tests/investigations	x	
Intervention/service provision	x	
Carer assessment(s)		
Other actions		

I agree that the information in the form is correct and consent to the further actions identified

Person signature	F Smith	Consent		Date	12-12-20
Carer signature	E Smith	Consent		Date	12-12-20
Assessor signature	**N Jones**			Date	12-12-20

Further notes/diagrams (using according to local protocols)

Appendix 4
What is abuse?

Please note this appendix is adapted from *Protecting Adults from Abuse and Neglect*, available at: www.tsab.org.uk/wp-content/uploads/2018/11/Safeguarding-Adults-Leaflet-English-Nov-2018-1.pdf (accessed 19 June 2019)

What is abuse?

Abuse may take the form of a single act or a series of acts, large or small, the impact of which 'adversely affects' the individual.

An adult may experience several types of abuse at the same time and there is often a lot of overlap between them, but it is also important that people should not restrict their view of what abuse and neglect can actually mean (taking advantage of someone is a common theme).

Discriminatory abuse

Including forms of harassment, slurs or similar treatment; because of race, gender and gender identity, age, disability, sexual orientation or religion.

Domestic abuse

Any incident or pattern of incidents of controlling, coercive, threatening behaviour, violence or abuse between those aged 16 or over who are, or have been, intimate partners or family members regardless of gender or sexuality. Including psychological, physical, sexual, financial, emotional abuse; so-called 'honour' based violence.

Financial or material abuse

Financial or material abuse can occur in isolation, but research has shown that where there are other forms of abuse, there is likely to be financial abuse occurring, although not always. Potential indicators include:

- Change in living conditions or lack of heating, clothing or food
- Inability to pay bills/unexplained shortage of money
- Unexplained loss/misplacement of financial documents
- The recent addition of authorised signers on signature cards.

Modern slavery

Encompasses slavery, human trafficking, forced labour and domestic servitude. Traffickers use whatever means to force individuals into a life of abuse and inhumane treatment.

Neglect and acts of omission

The failure of any person who has responsibility for the charge, care or custody of an adult at risk, to provide the amount and type of care that a reasonable person would be expected to provide. Neglect can be intentional or unintentional. Potential indicators include:

- Ignoring medical, emotional or physical care needs
- Failure to provide access to appropriate services
- Withholding the necessities of life, such as food and water.

Organisational abuse

Poor care within a care setting such as a hospital or care home that happens as a result of structures, policies, processes or practices in that organisation. Potential indicators include:

- deprived environmental conditions and lack of stimulation
- illegal confinement or restrictions
- inappropriate care of possessions, clothing and living area
- people left on a commode or a toilet for long periods of time
- people referred to, or spoken to with disrespect.

This may range from one-off incidents to ongoing ill treatment.

Physical abuse

Spotting the signs of physical abuse may not always be easy and sometimes people find it hard to believe that this type of abuse happens. Potential indicators including:

- black eyes, bruises, burns and cuts
- emotional distress
- restraint or grip markings
- unusual patterns of injury
- repeated trips to A&E.

Psychological abuse

Without the visible signs of physical abuse, psychological abuse can stay hidden for years. Psychological abuse can affect a person's thoughts and feelings as well as exert control over their life. Potential indicators include:

- exclusion from meaningful events or activities
- ignoring, imitating or mocking the person
- insulting the person and isolating the person
- name calling and yelling
- swearing and threatening
- threatening to take away something that is important.

Self-neglect

This covers a wide range of behaviours including neglecting to care for one's personal hygiene, health or surroundings, and hoarding. This could also involve refusal of services, treatment, assessments or intervention, which could potentially improve self-care or care of one's environment.

Sexual abuse and exploitation

This includes rape, indecent exposure, sexual harassment, inappropriate looking or touching, sexual teasing or innuendo, sexual photography, subjection to pornography or witnessing sexual acts. Sexual exploitation is the sexual abuse of an adult in exchange for attention, affection, food, drugs, shelter, protection, other basic necessities and/or money, and could be part of a seemingly consensual relationship. The person being exploited may believe their abuser is their friend, boyfriend or girlfriend. The abuser may:

- physically or verbally threaten the victim
- take indecent photographs of them and circulate to others
- be violent towards them or try to isolate them from friends and family.

Which adults are at risk of abuse?

Adult abuse can happen to anyone who is aged 18 or over. However, adults may be at 'greater risk' of abuse and neglect, less able to protect themselves and ask for help:

- if they have a physical, mental, sensory, learning or cognitive illness or disability
- linked to above; if they need assistance with everyday tasks
- if they rely on others for some kind of social care or health support
- if they are in receipt of care
- if they are informal carers, family and friends who provide care on an unpaid basis.

This list is not exhaustive.

Where does abuse occur?

Abuse can occur anywhere; examples include:

- care homes, day centres
- hospitals/health services
- in a carer's home, in the adult's own home (including online)
- public places
- supported living arrangements
- work, college or university.

Who are the perpetrators of abuse?

Anyone can be an abuser, examples include:
- family members/relatives (including partners)
- friends or neighbours
- other service users (including in care homes, hospitals, etc.)
- professionals (including paid carers)
- strangers
- unpaid carers, volunteers.

What not to do

- Don't promise to keep abuse a secret
- Don't alert the abuser; this might make matters worse and make it more difficult to help the person at risk
- Don't delay reporting abuse, report this straight away.

What happens next?

Every report of suspected abuse will be taken seriously.

The adult social care team and/or police will take steps to ensure the immediate safety of the adult at risk, and anyone else affected by the alleged abuse, including children.

The relevant agency will talk to the adult at risk (along with a suitable representative or advocate if necessary) to find out what is happening. They will work together with them to plan what is best to help keep the person safe, whilst respecting their views and wishes.

Please help to prevent further adult abuse

There is also lots of information available on the prevention of abuse, for example:

www.tsab.org.uk/key-information/prevention/

Find support in your area

Support can be accessed from a range of organisations based locally, this includes the statutory agencies such as the Local Authorities, Police and NHS, as well as numerous voluntary sector organisations.

Reproduced with permission from Teeswide Safeguarding Adults Board.

References

Andrews, C. and Roy, H.A. (2009) *The Roy Adaptation Model*, 3rd edition. Upper Saddle River, NJ: Pearson.

Arnstein, S.R. (1969) A ladder of citizen participation. *Journal of the American Planning Association*, **35(4)**: 216–24.

Banks, S. (2006) *Ethics and Values in Social Work*, 3rd edition. Basingstoke: Palgrave Macmillan.

Bate, A. (2017) *Early Intervention*. House of Commons Briefing Paper Number 7647, 26 June 2017. Available from https://researchbriefings.parliament.uk/ResearchBriefing/Summary/CBP-7647#fullreport (accessed 1 April 2019).

Benner, P. (1984) *From Novice to Expert*. California: Addison-Wesley.

Beresford, P. (2007) Service users do not want care navigators. *Community Care*, **(1668)**: 18.

Blaxter, M. (1990) *Health and Lifestyles*. London: Tavistock.

Blaxter, M. (2010) *Health (Key Concepts)*, 2nd edition. Cambridge: Polity Press.

Bradshaw, J. (1972) The concept of social need. *New Society*, **30**: 640–3.

Braye, S. and Preston-Shoot, M. (1995) *Empowering Practice in Social Care*. Buckingham: Open University Press.

Brophy, S., Snooks, H. and Griffiths, L. (2008) *Small-Scale Evaluation in Health: a practical guide*. London: Sage.

Care Quality Commission (2008) About us. Available from www.cqc.org.uk/about-us (accessed 1 April 2019).

Caris-Verhallen, W., Kerkstra, A. and Bensin, J. (1999) Non-verbal behaviour in nurse–elderly patient communication. *Journal of Advanced Nursing*, **29(4)**: 808–18.

Carnwell, R. and Buchanan, J. (2005) *Effective Practice in Health and Social Care: a partnership approach*. Maidenhead: Open University Press.

Carper, B.A. (1978) Fundamental patterns of knowing in nursing. *Advances in Nursing Science*, **1(1)**: 13–23.

Christensen, K. and Manthorpe, J. (2016) Personalised risk: new risk encounters facing migrant care workers. *Health, Risk and Society*, **18(3–4)**: 137–52.

Coverdale, G. (2009) Public health nursing. In: Thornbory, G. (ed.) *Public Health Nursing*. Chichester: Wiley-Blackwell.

Covey, S. (1989) *The Seven Habits of Highly Effective People*. London: Simon and Schuster.

Crinson, I. (2008) *Health Policy: a critical perspective*. London: Sage.

Dahlgren, G. and Whitehead, M. (1991) *Policies and Strategies to Promote Social Equity in Health*. Stockholm, Sweden: Institute for Futures Studies.

Dalton, C.C. and Gottlieb, L.N. (2003) The concept of readiness to change. *Journal of Advanced Nursing*, **42(2)**: 108–17.

Davis, A., Tschudin, V. and Tew, L. (2006) *Essentials of Teaching and Learning in Nursing Ethics: perspectives and methods*. London: Churchill Livingstone.

Department of Health (1997) *The New NHS: modern and dependable*. London: HMSO.

Department of Health (1998) *Modernising Social Services: promoting independence, improving protection, raising standards Cm. 4169*. London: HMSO.

Department of Health (2000) *Organisation with a Memory*. London: HMSO.

Department of Health (2001a) *The Expert Patient: a new approach to chronic disease management for the 21st century*. London: DH.

Department of Health (2001b) *National Service Framework for Older People*. London: DoH. Available from: https://assets.publishing.service.gov.uk/government/uploads/system/uploads/attachment_data/file/198033/National_Service_Framework_for_Older_People.pdf (accessed 10 April 2019).

Department of Health (2005) *Mental Capacity Act*. London: HMSO.

Department of Health (2006) *Dignity in Care*. London: Stationery Office.

Department of Health (2007) *Mental Health Act*. London: Stationery Office.

Department of Health (2008a) *High Quality Care for All*. London: Stationery Office.

Department of Health (2008b) *Health and Social Care Act*. London: Stationery Office.

Department of Health (2009) *Shaping the Future of Care Together*. London: HMSO.

Department of Health (2012a) *Health and Social Care Act*. London: HMSO.

Department of Health (2012b) *Informatics: the future*. London: Stationery Office.

Department of Health (2012c) *Liberating the NHS: no decision about me, without me*. London: HMSO.

Department of Health (2014a). *Care Act*. London: HMSO.

Department of Health (2014b) *Five Year Forward View.* London: HMSO.

Department of Health (2016) *Leading Change, Adding Value.* Available from: www.england.nhs.uk/wp-content/uploads/2016/05/nursing-framework.pdf (accessed 9 May 2019).

Dewey, J. (1933) *How We Think: a restatement of the relation of reflective thinking to the educative process.* Boston, MA: D.C. Heath & Co Publishers.

Dimond, B. (2005) *Legal Aspects of Nursing.* London: Longman.

Dominelli, L. (2007) The postmodern 'turn' in social work: the challenges of identity and equality. *Social Work and Society International Online Journal* **5(3)**. Available from: www.socwork.net/sws/article/view/144/513 (accessed 1 April 2019).

Donabedian, A. (1988) The quality of care: how can it be assessed? *Journal of the American Medical Association*, **260(12)**: 1743–8.

Dupré, C. (2011) What does dignity mean in a legal context? *The Guardian*, March 2011. Available from: www.theguardian.com/commentisfree/libertycentral/2011/mar/24/dignity-uk-europe-human-rights (accessed 14 May 2019)

Egan, G. (2002) *The Skilled Helper: a problem-management and opportunity-development approach to helping,* 7th edition. Pacific Grove, CA: Brooks/Cole.

Fawcett, B. and Karban, K. (2005) *Contemporary Mental Health: theory, policy and practice.* London: Routledge.

Forster, A., Lambley, R., Hardy, J. *et al.* (2009) Rehabilitation for older people in long-term care. *The Cochrane Database of Systematic Reviews*, Jan 21 (1): CD004294.

Fredriksson, L. and Lindström, U.A. (2002) Caring conversations – psychiatric patients' narratives about suffering. *Journal of Advanced Nursing*, **40(4)**: 396–404.

Frick, E., Riedner, C., Fegg, M. *et al.* (2006) A clinical interview assessing cancer patients' spiritual needs and preferences. *Cancer Care*, **15(3)**: 238–43.

Gambrill, E. (2012) *Critical Thinking in Clinical Practice: improving the quality of judgments and decisions*, 3rd edition. Hoboken, NJ: John Wiley & Sons, Inc.

Gibbs, G. (1988) *Learning by Doing: a guide to teaching and learning methods.* Oxford: Oxford Polytechnic.

Glasby, J. (2017) *Understanding Health and Social Care*, 3rd edition. Bristol: Policy Press.

Glasper, A. and Quiddington, J. (2009) Communication. In Glasper, A., McEwing, G. and Richardson, J. (eds). *Foundation Studies for Caring.* Basingstoke: Palgrave Macmillan, pp. 79–93.

Goddard, J. and Tavakoli, M. (2008) Efficiency and welfare implications of managed public sector hospital waiting lists. *European Journal of Operational Research,* **184**: 778–92.

Gramsci, A. (1971) *Selections from the Prison Notebooks*. London: New Left Books.

Greenhalgh, T. (2000) *How to Read a Paper: the basics of evidence-based medicine.* London: BMJ Books.

Gubbay, J. (1997) Power: Concepts and Research. In Gubbay, J., Middleton, C. and Ballard, C. (eds) *The Student's Companion to Sociology*. Oxford: Blackwell, pp. 152–61.

Guo, K.L. (2008) DECIDE: a decision-making model for more effective decision making by health care managers. *Health Care Management*, **27(2)**: 118–27.

Hambridge, K. and McEwing, G. (2009) Care of the adult – surgical. In Glasper, A., McEwing, G. and Richardson, J. (eds) *Foundation Studies for Caring*. Basingstoke: Palgrave Macmillan, pp. 440–76.

Harrison, G. and Melville, R. (2010) *Rethinking Social Work in a Global World*. London: Palgrave Macmillan.

Hatton, K. (2008) *New Directions in Social Work Practice*. Exeter: Learning Matters.

Hayes, S. and Llewellyn, A. (2008) *Fundamentals of Nursing Care: a textbook for students of nursing and health care*. Exeter: Reflect Press.

Henderson, V. (1960) *Basic Principles of Nursing Care*. Geneva: International Council for Nurses.

HM Government (2018) *Working Together to Safeguard Children: a guide to inter-agency working to safeguard and promote the welfare of children*. Available from: www. assets.publishing.service.gov.uk/government/uploads/system/uploads/attachment_ data/file/779401/Working_Together_to_Safeguard-Children.pdf (accessed 19 June 2019).

Hockley, J. and Clark, D. (2002) *Palliative Care for Older People in Care Homes*. Buckingham: Open University Press.

Hogston, R. (2007) Managing nursing care. In: Hogston, R. and Marjoram B.A. (eds) *Foundations of Nursing Practice: leading the way,* 3rd edition. Basingstoke: Palgrave Macmillan, pp. 2–25.

Hogston, R. (2011) Managing nursing care. In: Hogston, R. and Marjoram, B. (eds) *Foundations of Nursing Practice: themes, concepts and frameworks*, 4th edition. Basingstoke: Palgrave Macmillan, pp. 2–21.

Howatson-Jones, I., Roberts, S. and Standing, M. (2015) *Patient Assessment and Care Planning in Nursing*. Exeter: Learning Matters.

Hudson, B. (2002) Interprofessionality in health and social care: the Achilles' heel of partnership. *Journal of Interprofessional Care*, **16(1)**: 7–17.

Huycke, L. and All, A. (2000) Quality in health care and ethical principles. *Journal of Advanced Nursing*, **32(3)**: 562–71.

Illich, I. (1976) *Limits to Medicine: the expropriation of health*. London: Marion Boyars.

Johns, C. (2004) *Becoming a Reflective Practitioner*. Oxford: Blackwell.

Jones, D.P.H. (2003) *Communicating with Vulnerable Children: A Guide for Practitioners*. London: Royal College of Psychiatrists.

Kaplan, R. and Norton, D. (1996) *The Balanced Scorecard: Translating Strategy into Action*. Harvard: Harvard Business School Press.

Kendall, J. (1992) Fighting back: Promoting emancipatory nursing actions. *Advances in Nursing Science*, **15(2)**: 1–15.

King, R. and Raynes, N. (1968) An operational measure of inmate management in residential institutions. *Journal of Social Sciences and Medicine*, **2**: 41–53.

King's Fund (2017) *What are the priorities for health and social care?* London: The King's Fund. Available at: www.kingsfund.org.uk/publications/what-are-priorities-health-and-social-care (accessed 10 April 2019).

Kitwood, T. (1993) Towards a theory of dementia care – the interpersonal process. *Ageing and Society*, **13(1)**: 51–67.

Klein, R. (2005) *The Politics of the NHS*, 2nd edition. Harlow: Longman.

Kleinman, A. (1988) *The Illness Narratives: suffering, healing and the human condition*. New York: Basic Books.

Law, M. (2000) Strategies for implementing evidence-based practice in early intervention. *Infants and Young Children*, **13(2)**: 32–40.

Law Society (2015) *Deprivation of liberty: a practical guide*. Available from: www.lawsociety.org.uk/support-services/advice/articles/deprivation-of-liberty/ (accessed 9 May 2019).

Lee-Treweek, G. (1997) Women, resistance and care: an ethnographic study of nursing work. *Work, Employment and Society*, **11(1)**: 47–65.

Leininger, M. and McFarland, M. (2005) *Culture Care Diversity and Universality: a worldwide nursing theory*, 2nd edition. Burlington, MA: Jones & Bartlett Learning.

Lindberg, J.B., Hunter, M.L. and Kruszewski, A.Z. (1990) *Introduction to Nursing: concepts, issues and opportunities*. Philadelphia, PA: Lippincott.

Llewellyn, A., Agu, L. and Mercer, D. (2015) *Sociology for Social Workers*, 2nd edition. Cambridge: Polity Press.

Lord Laming (2009) *The Protection of Children in England: a progress report*. London: HMSO. Available from: https://assets.publishing.service.gov.uk/government/uploads/system/uploads/attachment_data/file/328117/The_Protection_of_Children_in_England.pdf (accessed 4 June 2019).

Macionis, J. and Plummer, K. (2012) *Sociology: a global introduction*, 5th edition. Harlow: Prentice Hall.

Marquis, B. and Huston, C. (2008) *Leadership Roles and Management Functions in Nursing: theory and application*, 6th edition. Philadelphia, PA: Lippincott Williams & Wilkins.

Martell, L. (2010) *The Sociology of Globalization*. Cambridge: Polity Press.

Maslow, A. (1962) *Motivation and Personality*. New York: Harper.

McDonald, C. (2006) *Challenging Social Work: the context of practice*. London: Palgrave Macmillan.

McGinnis, E. (2009) Crisis intervention. In Lindsay, T. (ed.) *Social Work Intervention*. Exeter: Learning Matters, pp. 35–51.

Menzies, I.E.P. (1960) Nurses under stress: a social system functioning as a defence against anxiety. *International Nursing Review*, **1(6)**: 9–16.

Milner, J. and O'Byrne, P. (2009) *Assessment in Social Work*, 3rd edition. London: Palgrave Macmillan.

Moon, G. and Gillespie, R. (1995) *Society and Health: an introduction to social science for health professionals*. London: Routledge.

Moore, R. (2009) Technology can help nurses improve patient care. *Nursing Times*, 14 May 2009. Available from www.nursingtimes.net/technology-can-help-nurses-improve-patient-care/5001545.article (accessed 9 May 2019).

Morgan, C. and Hutchinson, G. (2010) The social determinants of psychosis in migrant and ethnic minority populations: a public health tragedy. *Psychological Medicine*, **40(5)**: 705–9.

Muir Gray, J.A. (1997) *Evidence-based Healthcare: how to make health policy and management decisions*. London: Churchill Livingstone.

National Institute for Clinical Excellence (2002) *Principles for Best Practice in Clinical Audit*. Abingdon: Radcliffe Medical Press Ltd. Available at www.nice.org.uk/media/default/About/what-we-do/Into-practice/principles-for-best-practice-in-clinical-audit.pdf (accessed 3 April 2019).

National Institute for Health and Care Excellence (2016) VitalPAC for assessing vital signs of patients in hospital. Available at www.nice.org.uk/advice/mib79 (accessed 10 May 2019).

Nettleton, S. (2013) *The Sociology of Health and Illness*. Cambridge: Polity.

Neuman, M. (1995) *A Developing Discipline*. New York: National League for Nursing Press.

NHS England (2015) *The NHS Constitution for England 2015*. London: HMSO. Available from: www.gov.uk/government/publications/the-nhs-constitution-for-england/the-nhs-constitution-for-england (accessed 10 May 2019).

NHS England (2017) *Next Steps on the NHS Five year Forward View*. London: HMSO. Available from: www.england.nhs.uk/wp-content/uploads/2017/03/NEXT-STEPS-ON-THE-NHS-FIVE-YEAR-FORWARD-VIEW.pdf (accessed 3 April 2019).

NHS Executive (1999) *Clinical Governance: quality in the new NHS*. London: Department of Health. Available from: https://webarchive.nationalarchives.gov.uk/20120510094745/http://www.dh.gov.uk/prod_consum_dh/groups/dh_digitalassets/@dh/@en/documents/digitalasset/dh_4012043.pdf (accessed 9 May 2019).

NHS Institute for Innovation and Improvement (2011) *Plan, Do, Study, Act (PDSA)*. Available from https://webarchive.nationalarchives.gov.uk/20121108074656/http://www.institute.nhs.uk/quality_and_service_improvement_tools/quality_and_service_improvement_tools/plan_do_study_act.html (accessed 3 April 2019).

Nursing and Midwifery Council (2018a) *The Code: professional standards of practice and behaviour for nurses, midwives and nursing associates*. London: NMC. Available from: www.nmc.org.uk/standards/code/ (accessed 14 May 2019).

Nursing and Midwifery Council (2018b) *Future Nurse: standards of proficiency for registered nurses*. London: NMC. Available from: www.nmc.org.uk/standards/standards-for-nurses/standards-of-proficiency-for-registered-nurses (accessed 10 April 2019).

Office for National Statistics (2019) *Internet Users, UK: 2019*. London: HMSO. Available from: www.ons.gov.uk/businessindustryandtrade/itandinternetindustry/bulletins/internetusers/2019#still-a-difference-in-internet-use-between-men-and-women-in-older-age-groups (accessed 18 June 2019).

Oliviere, D., Hargreaves, R. and Monroe, B. (eds) (1998) *Good Practice in Palliative Care*. Aldershot: Ashgate.

Olshansky, E. (2017) Social determinants of health: the role of nursing. *American Journal of Nursing*, **117(12)**: 11.

Parry-Jones, B. and Soulsby, J. (2001) Needs-led assessment: the challenges and the reality. *Health and Social Care in the Community*, **9(6)**: 414–28.

Parsons, T. (1951) *The Social System*. London: Routledge and Kegan Paul.

Patterson, E. (1998) The philosophy and physics of holistic health care: spiritual healing and a workable interpretation. *Journal of Advanced Nursing*, **27(2)**: 287–93.

Peplau, H.E. (1952) *Interpersonal Relations in Nursing: a conceptual frame of reference for psychodynamic nursing*. New York: G. P. Putnum's Sons.

Picker Institute (2009) *Using Patient Feedback – a practical guide*. Available from: www.nhssurveys.org/Filestore/documents/QIFull.pdf? (accessed 10 May 2019).

Pollock, A. and Talbot-Smith, A. (2006) *The New NHS: a guide to its funding, organisation and accountability*. London: Routledge.

Prime Minister's Commission (2010) *Front Line Care: the future of nursing and midwifery in England*. London: HMSO.

Public Health England (2017a) *Living Well in Older Years*. Available at: www.gov.uk/government/publications/better-mental-health-jsna-toolkit/7-living-well-in-older-years (accessed 10 April 2019).

Public Health England (2017b) *Health Profile for England: 2017*. Available from: www.gov.uk/government/publications/health-profile-for-england (accessed 3 April 2019).

Public Health England (2018) *Healthy child programme 0 to 19: health visitor and school nurse commissioning*. Available from: www.gov.uk/government/publications/healthy-child-programme-0-to-19-health-visitor-and-school-nurse-commissioning (accessed 3 April 2019).

Quilter, R.N., Wheeler, S. and Windt, J. (1993) *Telephone Triage: theory, practice and protocol development*. New York: Delmar.

Rapaport, J., Manthorpe, J., Moriarty, J. *et al.* (2005) Advocacy and people with learning disabilities in the UK: how can local funders find value for money? *Journal of Intellectual Disabilities*, **9(94)**: 299–319.

Richardson, J. (2009) Culture. In Glasper, A., McEwing, G. and Richardson, J. (eds) *Foundation Studies for Caring*. Basingstoke: Palgrave Macmillan, pp. 94–103.

Roper, N., Logan, W. and Tierney, A. (2000) *The Roper-Logan-Tierney Model of Nursing Based on Activities of Living*. Edinburgh: Churchill Livingstone.

Rosenberg, W. and Donald, A. (1995) Evidence based medicine: an approach to clinical problem-solving. *BMJ*, **310**: 1122–6.

Rourke, A.J. and Coleman, K.S. (eds) (2011) *Pedagogy Leads Technology: online learning and teaching in higher education: new technologies, new pedagogies*. Champaign, IL: Common Ground Publishing, LLC.

Routasalo, P. and Isola, A. (1998) Touching by skilled nurses in elderly care. *Scandinavian Journal of Caring Sciences*, **12(3)**: 170–8.

Royal College of Nursing (2011) *A Decisive Decade – mapping the future NHS workforce* by James Buchan and Ian Seccombe. Available from: www.rcn.org.uk/-/media/royal-college-of-nursing/documents/publications/2011/july/pub-004158.pdf (accessed 5 June 2019).

Royal College of Nursing (2012) *This is Nursing – Northern region*. Available from: www.rcn.org.uk/professional-development/publications/pub-004257 (accessed 5 June 2019).

Royal College of Nursing (2017) *Understanding Benchmarking*. Available from: www.rcn.org.uk/professional-development/publications/pub-006333 (accessed 5 June 2019)

Sackett, D.L., Rosenberg, W.M., Muir Gray, J.A. *et al.* (1996) Evidence based medicine: what it is and what it isn't. *British Medical Journal*, **312(7023)**: 71–2.

Sainsbury Centre for Mental Health (2002) *Breaking the Circles of Fear.* Available from: www.centreformentalhealth.org.uk/sites/default/files/breaking_the_circles_of_fear. pdf (accessed 18 June 2019).

Schön, D.A. (1984) *The Reflective Practitioner: how professionals think in action.* New York: Basic Books.

Seedhouse, D. (2009) *Ethics: the heart of health care*, 3rd edition. Wiley: Chichester.

Shannon, C.E. and Weaver, W. (1949) *A Mathematical Model of Communication.* Urbana, IL: University of Illinois Press.

Shin, K.R., Lee, J.H., Ha, J.Y. and Kim, K.H. (2006) Critical thinking dispositions in baccalaureate nursing students. *Journal of Advanced Nursing*, **56(2)**: 182–9.

Smale, G.G. and Tuson, G., with Biehal, N. and Marsh, P. (eds) (1993) *Empowerment, Assessment, Care Management and the Skilled Worker.* London: HMSO.

Social Care Institute for Excellence (2013) *Dignity in Care.* SCIE Guide 15. Available from: www.scie.org.uk/publications/guides/guide15/index.asp (accessed 4 April 2019).

Standing, M. (2017) *Clinical Judgement and Decision Making in Nursing*, 3rd edition. London: Learning Matters.

Stark, J. (1995) Critical thinking. Taking the road less traveled. *Nursing*, **25(11)**: 52–6.

Stickley (2011) From SOLER to SURETY for effective non-verbal communication. *Nurse Education in Practice*, **11(6)**: 395–8.

Stockwell, F. (1972) *The Unpopular Patient.* London: Royal College of Nursing.

Sully, P. and Dallas, J. (2010) *Essential Communication Skills for Nursing and Midwifery*, 2nd edition. Mosby Elsevier.

Sutton, C. (2006) *Helping Families with Troubled Children: a preventive approach*, 2nd edition. Chichester: Wiley.

Tan, S. and Goonawardene, N. (2017) Internet health information seeking and the patient–physician relationship: a systematic review. *Journal of Medical Internet Research*, **19(1)**: 73–87.

Thomas, D. and Woods, H. (2003) *Working with People with Learning Disabilities: theory to practice.* London: Jessica Kingsley Publishers.

Thompson, N. (2005) *Understanding Social Work: preparing for practice*, 2nd edition. Basingstoke: Palgrave Macmillan.

Thompson, N. (2007) *Power and Empowerment.* Oxford: Russell House Publishers.

Thompson, C. and Dowding, D. (eds) (2009) *Essential Decision Making and Clinical Judgement for Nurses*. Edinburgh: Churchill Livingstone.

Thompson, N. and Thompson, S. (2008) *The Social Work Companion*. London: Palgrave.

Tones, K. and Green, J. (2004) *Health Promotion: planning and strategies*. London: Sage.

Tutton, E. (1991) Breaking the mould. In McMahon, R. and Pearson, A. (eds) *Nursing as Therapy*. Suffolk: Chapman and Hall, pp. 169–200.

Walker, E. and Dewar, B. (2001) How do we facilitate carers' involvement in decision making? *Journal of Advanced Nursing*, **34(3)**: 329–37.

Weber, M. (1976) *The Protestant Ethic and the Spirit of Capitalism*. London: Allen & Unwin.

Whittington, C. (2003) *Learning for Collaborative Practice with other Professions and Agencies: a study to inform the development of the degree in social work*. London: Department of Health.

Winkleby, M., Feighery, E., Dunn, M. *et al.* (2004) Effects of an advocacy intervention to reduce smoking among teenagers. *Archive of Pediatric Adolescence Medicine*, **158**: 269–75.

World Health Organization (1984) *Report on the Working Group on Concepts and Principles of Health Promotion*. Copenhagen: WHO.

World Health Organization/United Nations Children's Fund (2009) *Who Child Growth Standards and the Identification of Severe Acute Malnutrition in Infants and Children: a joint statement*. Available from: https://apps.who.int/iris/bitstream/handle/10665/44129/9789241598163_eng.pdf?ua=1 (accessed 10 May 2019).

Wu, S., Chao Yu, Y., Yang, C. and Che, H. (2005) Decision-making tree for women considering hysterectomy. *Journal of Advanced Nursing*, **51(4)**: 361–8.

Young, C. (1987) Intuition and nursing process. *Holistic Nursing Practice*, **1(3)**: 52–62.

Index

Bold indicates main entry